M00268258

Pulmonary Vein Electrograms

Self Assessment

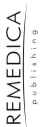

REMEDICA

p u b l i s h i n g

LONDON • CHICAGO

Pulmonary Vein Electrograms is intended to accompany *Pulmonary Vein Recordings: A Practical Guide to the Mapping and Ablation of Atrial Fibrillation*, by Laurent Macle.

Published by the Remedica Group
Remedica Publishing, 32–38 Osnaburgh Street, London, NW1 3ND, UK
Remedica Inc, Civic Opera Building, 20 North Wacker Drive, Suite 1642, Chicago, IL, 60606, USA

Email: books@remedica.com
www.remedica.com/books

Publisher: Andrew Ward
In-house editor: Cath Harris
Printed in Canada

© January 2004 Remedica Publishing

ISBN 1 901346 55 2

British Library Cataloguing in-Publication Data
A catalogue record for this book is available from the British Library.

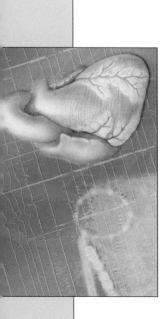

Pulmonary Vein Electrograms

Self Assessment

Christophe Scavée, MD
Université Catholique de Louvain, Belgium

Rukshen Weerasooriya, BMed Sc, MBBS, FRACP
Royal Perth Hospital, University of Western Australia, Australia

Laurent Macle, MD
Montreal Heart Institute, Canada

Foreword by:
Michel Haïssaguerre, MD
Hôpital Cardiologique du Haut-Lévêque
Bordeaux-Pessac, France

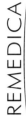

REMEDICA
publishing

LONDON • CHICAGO

ACKNOWLEDGMENTS

We remember our fellowship in Bordeaux with great fondness.

We are deeply indebted to Michel Haïssaguerre, Pierre Jais, Meleze Hocini, and Dipen Shah for being such wonderful teachers of cardiac electrophysiology and, in particular, for greatly enriching our understanding of pulmonary vein electrograms.

We are also grateful for the many excellent questions posed by electrophysiologists from around the world visiting the Hôpital Cardiologique du Haut-Lévêque in Bordeaux, France, during our fellowship, as these questions served as a stimulus for us to commence this book.

Christophe Scavée, Université Catholique de Louvain, Belgium
Rukshen Weerasooriya, Royal Perth Hospital, University of Western Australia, Australia
Laurent Macle, Montreal Heart Institute, Canada
November, 2003

TABLE OF CONTENTS

Foreword	ii
Recording settings	iii
Abbreviations	iv
Cases	1
Appendix 1	270
Appendix 2	272
Appendix 3	274
Appendix 4	276
Appendix 5	278

FOREWORD

Catheter ablation of pulmonary veins (PVs) guided by circumferential mapping of PV signals is a complex procedure with a potentially steep learning curve. A good working understanding of PV electrograms is an important step in reducing this learning curve, and helps the operator to undertake PV ablation procedures in an efficient and timely manner. During the past few years, the ablation approach to atrial fibrillation has changed quite dramatically – from linear ablation first in the right and then in the left atrium, to focal ablation within PVs, and finally to the current strategy of systematic PV disconnection as the first step of atrial fibrillation ablation.

It is feasible, and should be the aim of all electrophysiologists undertaking PV isolation, to achieve disconnection in 100% of veins using irrigated tip catheters and a power limitation. Since the recognition of PV stenosis as a potential complication, very ostial ablation has been insisted upon. This is possible in all veins, except in some parts where a slight encroachment is required to achieve adequate catheter stability. As long as ablation is carried out very ostially and with controlled power, the risk of PV stenosis is low (<1%). Correct interpretation of PV versus superimposed surrounding signals enables the electrophysiologist to minimize the amount of ablative energy.

This book will assist students of electrophysiology and those electrophysiologists commencing PV ablation to gain a better understanding of PV electrograms using a simple question and answer, case-oriented approach. The electrograms have been carefully chosen by Drs Scavée, Weerasooriya, and Macle to demonstrate and reinforce important points.

Michel Haïssaguerre
Hôpital Cardiologique du Haut-Lévêque,
Bordeaux-Pessac, France

RECORDING SETTINGS

Electrogram recording settings

- LASSO™ catheter[a]   0.45 mV/cm

- RF catheter   0.115 mV/cm

- CS catheter   0.45 mV/cm

Recording and ablation materials

- A dual-recording system (LabSystem™ Duo™; Bard Electrophysiology, MA, USA) was used to obtain all of the recordings in this book.

- A 65-cm sheath (Preface™; Biosense Webster, CA, USA) was used for transseptal puncture.

- The ablation catheter was a 5-mm irrigated-tip catheter coupled to an automatic triggered pump (Coolflow; Cordis Webster, USA) and a Stockert-70 Generator (Biosense Webster, CA, USA).

- PV recordings were made using a 15 mm or 20 mm LASSO™ catheter (Biosense Webster, CA, USA).

- A quadripolar 6F steerable catheter (Xtrem™; Ela Medical, France) was used for coronary sinus recordings.

Ablation settings

- The power setting was 30 W for ostial ablation of the LSPV, RSPV, and RIPV, and 25 W for the LIPV because of the higher risk of PV stenosis in this vein. The temperature limit was set at 50°C during all applications, but was rarely reached because of the use of an externally irrigated ablation catheter (Thermo-Cool; Cordis-Webster).

[a]LASSO™ is a trademark of Biosense Webster.

ABBREVIATIONS

A	atrial activity	PV	pulmonary vein
AFIB	atrial fibrillation	PVP	pulmonary vein potential
AP	antero-posterior	RA	right atrium
CS	coronary sinus	RF	radiofrequency
ECG	electrocardiogram	RIPV	right inferior pulmonary vein
LA	left atrium	RPV	right pulmonary vein
LAA	left atrial appendage	RSPV	right superior pulmonary vein
LIPV	left inferior pulmonary vein	S	stimulus artifact
LPV	left pulmonary vein	V	ventricular activity
LSPV	left superior pulmonary vein		

Cases

CASE 1 PART 1

- This tracing is from an LIPV during CS pacing prior to any ablation (the LASSO™ shaft is at the top of the vein).

  Where is the ablation target?

Paper speed 100 mm/s

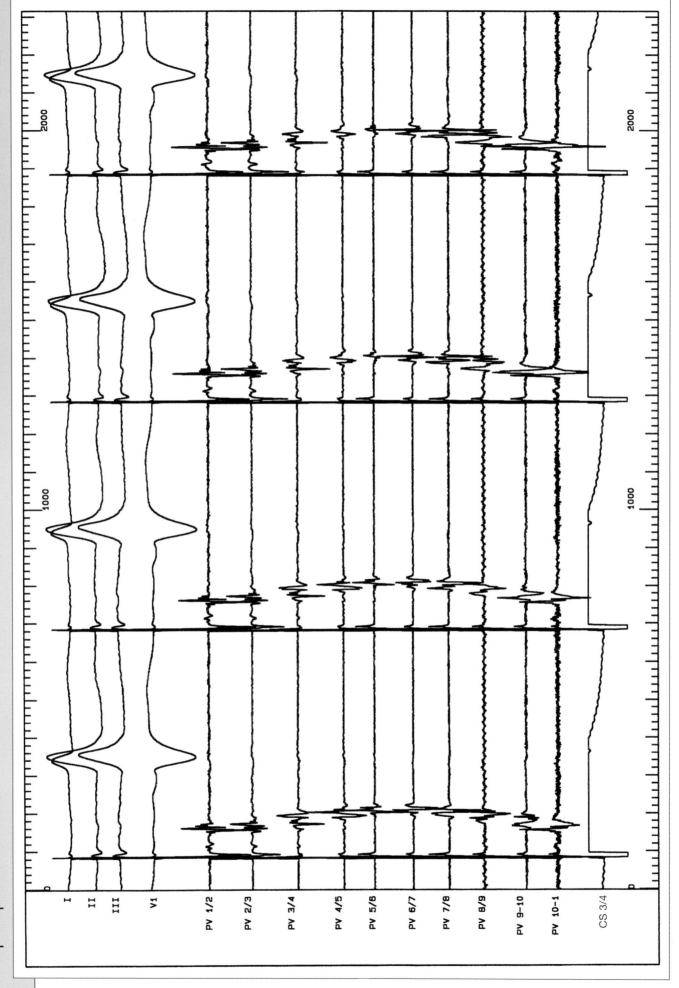

CASE 1 PART 2

- When the LASSO shaft is at the top of the left-sided veins, poles 1–5 represent the anterior wall and poles 6–10 represent the posterior wall. The ablation target is at pole 1 at the top of the vein: the PV activity is earliest here (✱ and arrows) and has a clear activation sequence, which is sometimes referred to as a "cascade" of PVPs.

Paper speed 100 mm/s

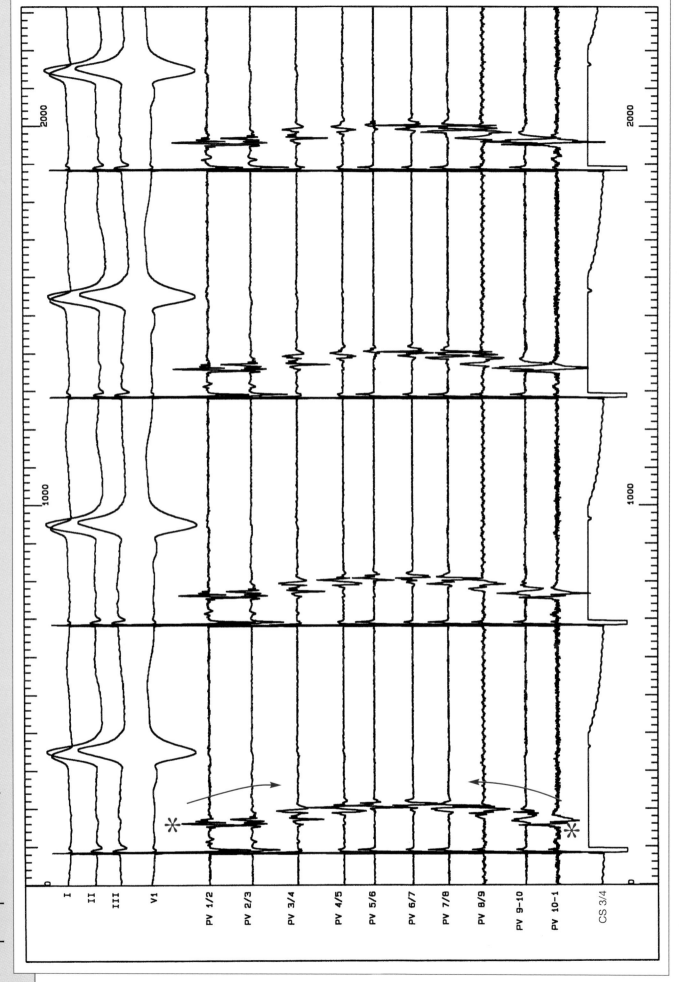

CASE 2 PART 1

- This tracing is from an LIPV during CS pacing (the LASSO shaft is at the top of the vein).

  Where is the ablation target?

Paper speed 100 mm/s

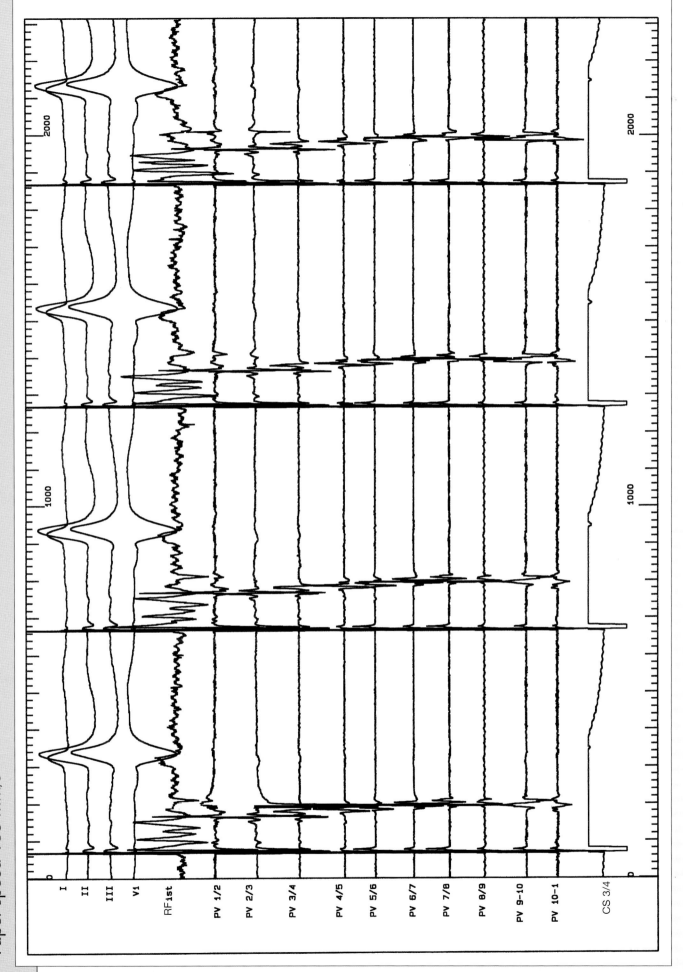

CASE 2 PART 2

- The mapping catheter displays an ideal ablation site, with fractionated activity bridging the interval between the pacing artifact and the earliest PVP (box). The target site is at LASSO pole 2 at the top anterior part of the vein, as this shows the earliest activation (dotted line) with polarity reversal. Note that there is a touching artifact (arrow) as the ablation catheter is directly on pole 2. In order to remove the risk of charring and coagulum formation on the LASSO catheter, it is advisable to withdraw the mapping catheter to a more ostial position prior to ablation.

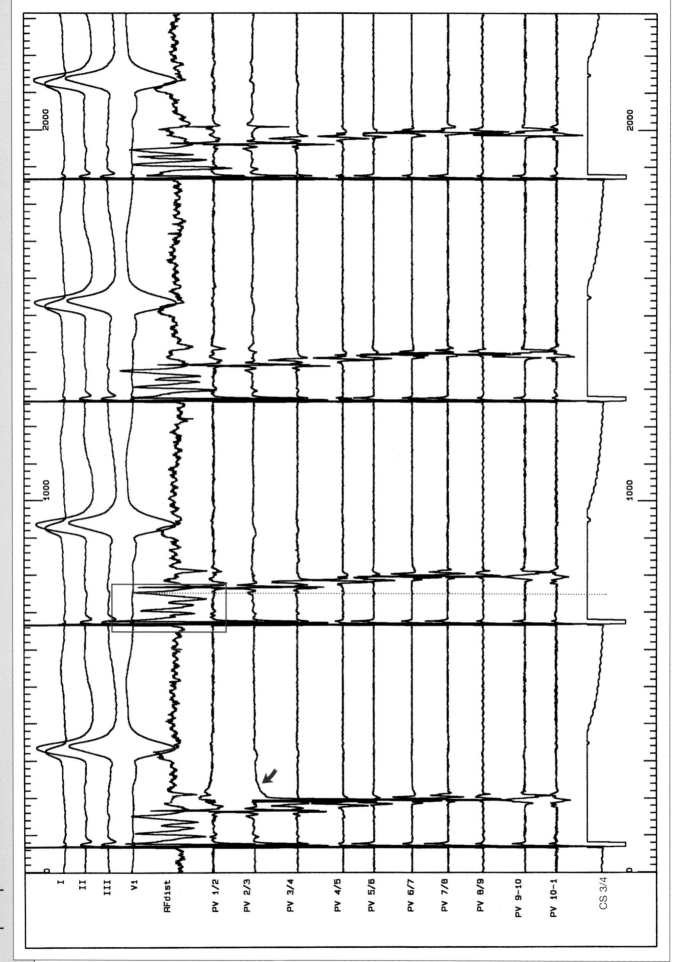

Paper speed 100 mm/s

CASE 3 PART 1

- After disconnecting all four PVs, it is important to check each for conduction recovery, beginning with the first vein ablated. This tracing is from an RSPV after ablation (the LASSO pole is at the top of the vein).

  Is the vein still disconnected?

Paper speed 100 mm/s

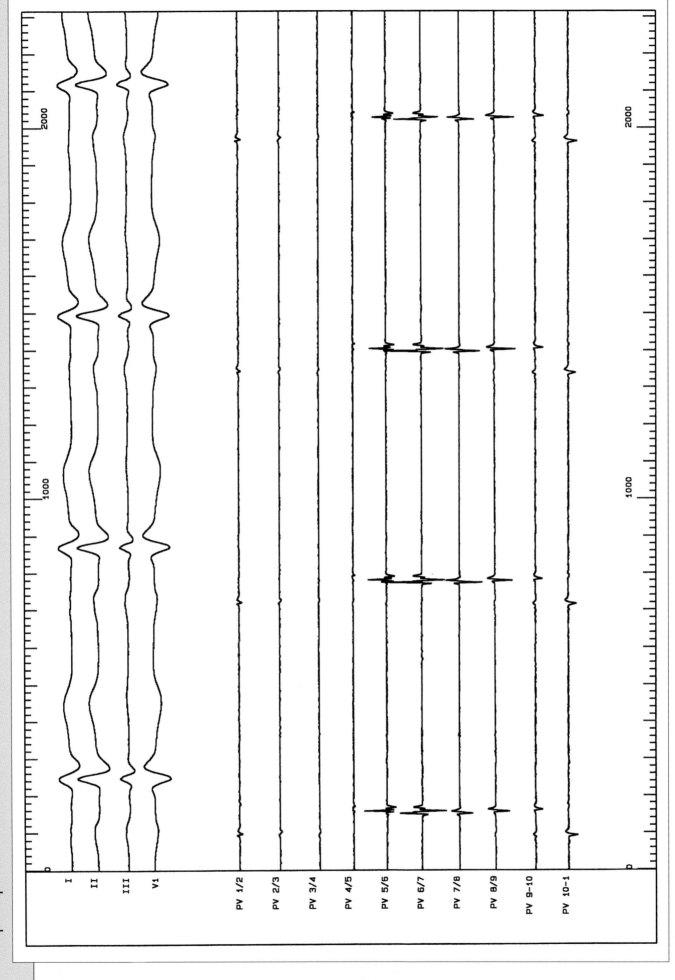

CASE 3 PART 2

- Because this is a right-sided PV with the LASSO shaft at the top of the vein, poles 1–5 are recording activity from the posterior part of the vein, while poles 6–10 are recording activity from the anterior part. There is conduction recovery with a PVP clearly visible on poles 6–10, corresponding to the bottom and anterior part of the vein (solid line).

  Bipoles 6/7 and 7/8 display the earliest signals and polarity reversal. The ablation target is pole 7 at the anterior part of the vein. Atrial far-field signals (A) can be seen, which probably represent LA far-field as the signal is late within the sinus P wave (dotted lines).

Paper speed 100 mm/s

CASE 3 PART 3

- After further ablation in the same vein, the following tracing is recorded (the LASSO shaft is at the top of the vein).

Is further energy delivery required?

Paper speed 100 mm/s

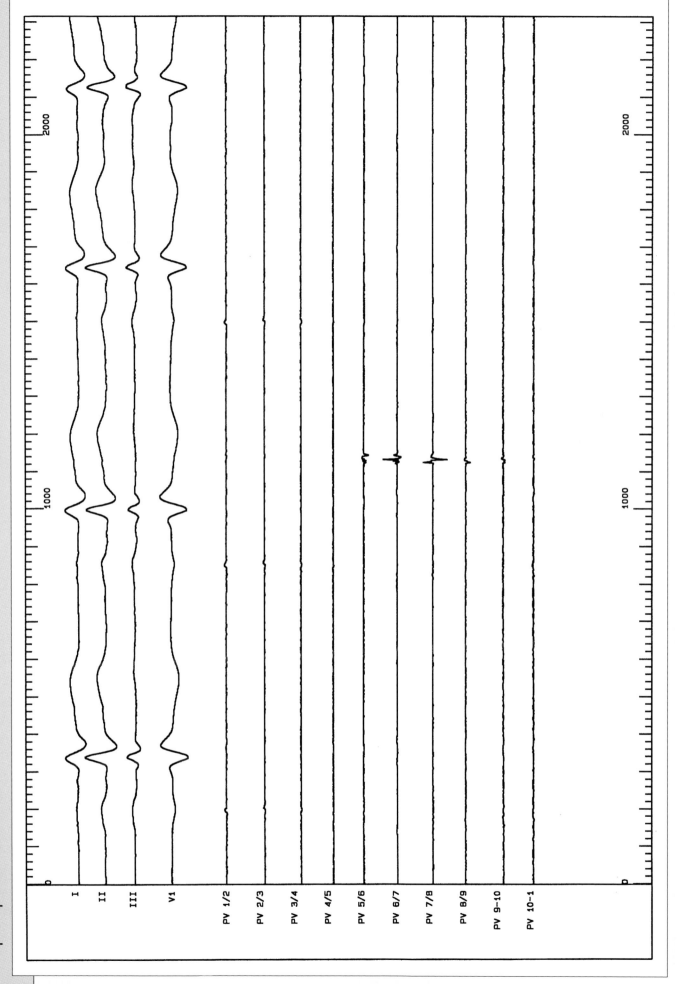

CASE 3 PART 4

- This is an example of dissociated PV activity (PVP) in the bottom and anterior part of this RSPV. The vein is disconnected and further energy delivery is not required. Note that the activation sequence is similar to preablation, with polarity reversal at LASSO bipoles 6/7 and 7/8. The posterior LA far-field signal is recorded on poles 1–3.

Paper speed 100 mm/s

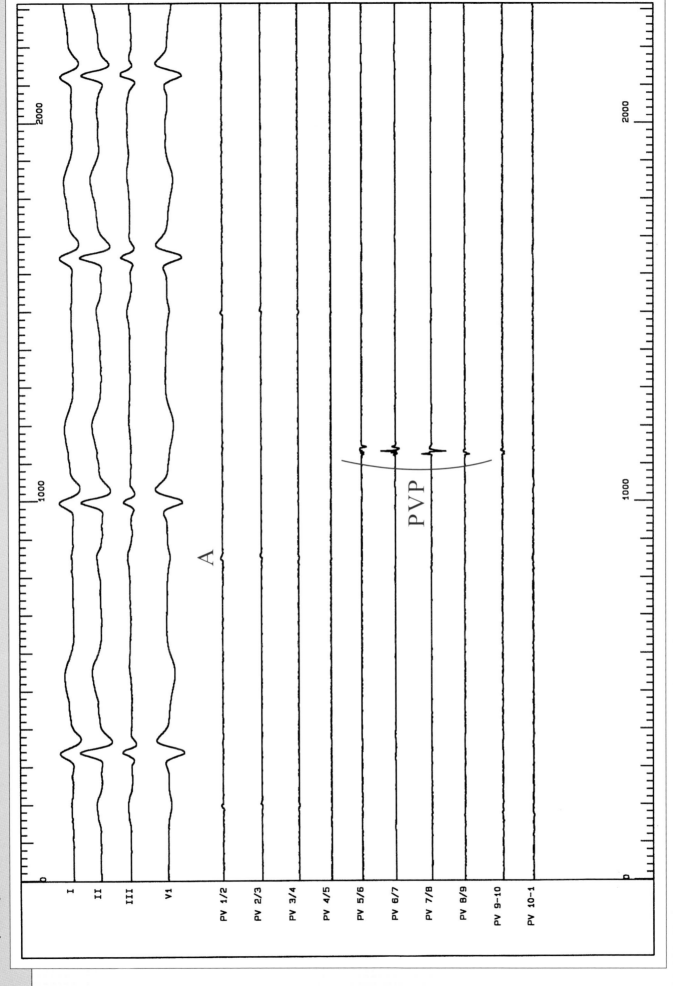

CASE 4 PART 1

- A patient previously ablated for AFIB presents to the electrophysiology laboratory following symptomatic AFIB recurrence. This tracing shows electrical activity recorded in the LIPV using the LASSO catheter prior to ablation (the LASSO shaft is at the top of the vein).

  What is your interpretation of the tracing?

  Would pacing be useful?

  (Paper speed 50 mm/s – turn the page for 100 mm/s.)

Paper speed 50 mm/s

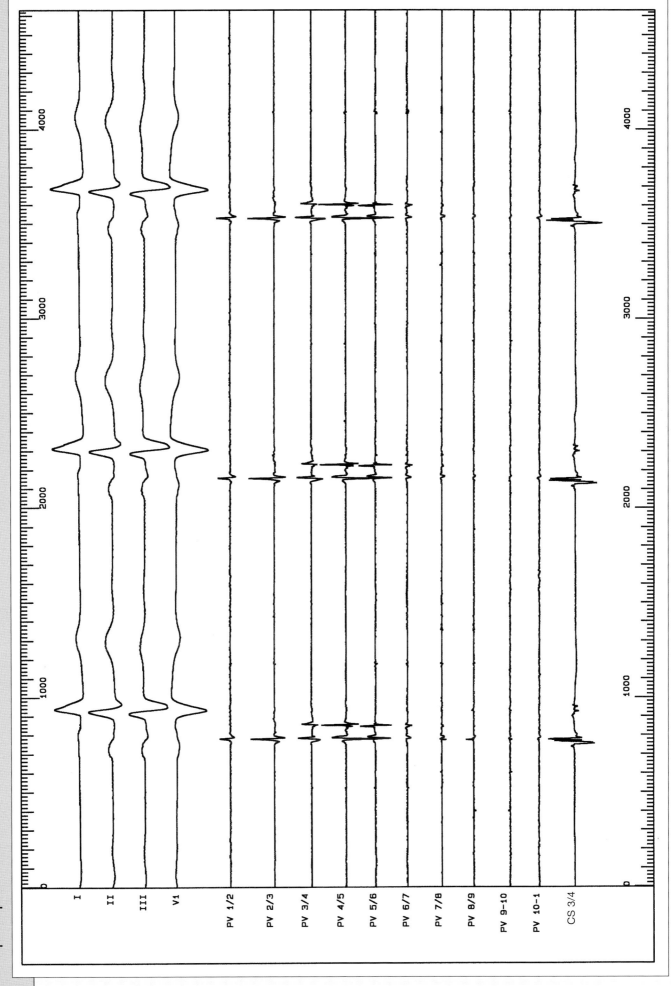

CASE 4 PART 2

- The same tracing at 100 mm/s.

Paper speed 100 mm/s

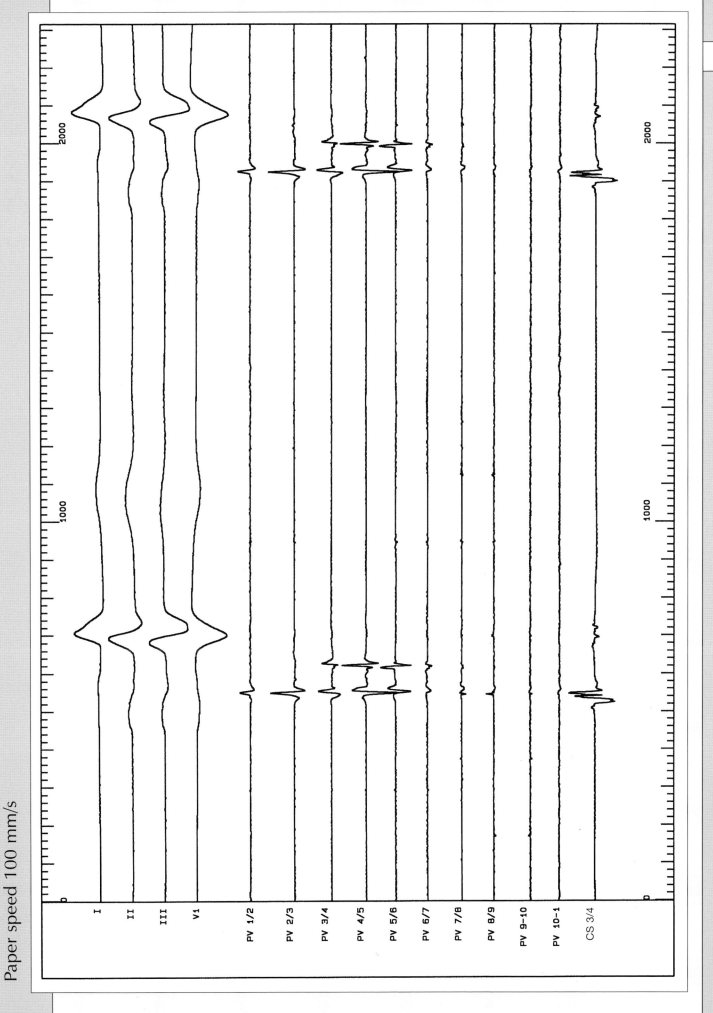

CASE 4 PART 3

- The patient is currently in sinus rhythm. The tracing shows a typical "recovered vein" pattern, with delayed PVPs visible even without the need for pacing (✱). This is presumably because the previous ablation slowed conduction into the vein, but did not completely abolish it. Pacing may be useful in determining the earliest site of breakthrough. In this case, the atrial far-field signal (A) is clearly distinct from the PVPs.

Note polarity reversal at LASSO bipoles 4/5 and 5/6, indicating that the ablation target is at the bottom of this vein. Ablation of recovered PV activity is usually relatively easy as there are limited breakthroughs – often, a single application is sufficient to disconnect the vein.

Paper speed 100 mm/s

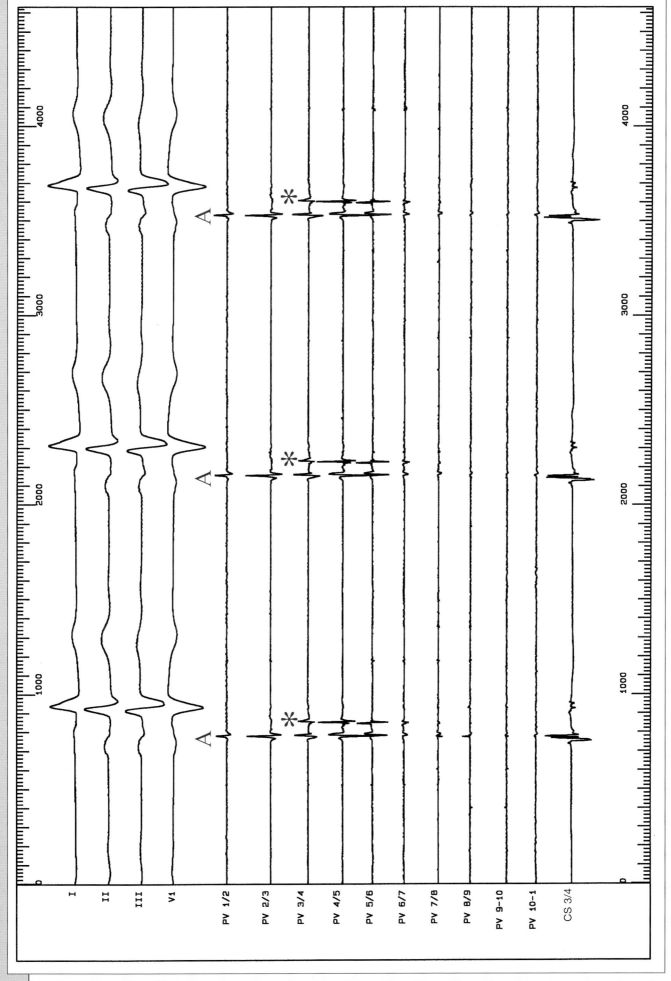

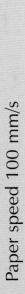

CASE 4 PART 4

- Following ablation and disconnection of the LIPV in the same patient, the LASSO was placed in the LSPV (the LASSO shaft is at the top of the vein) and this tracing was obtained.

What is your interpretation?

(Paper speed 50 mm/s – turn the page for 100 mm/s.)

Paper speed 50 mm/s

I
II
III
V1

PV 1/2
PV 2/3
PV 3/4
PV 4/5
PV 5/6
PV 6/7
PV 7/8
PV 8/9
PV 9-10
PV 10-1
CS 3/4

1000 2000 3000 4000

25

- The same tracing at 100 mm/s.

Paper speed 100 mm/s

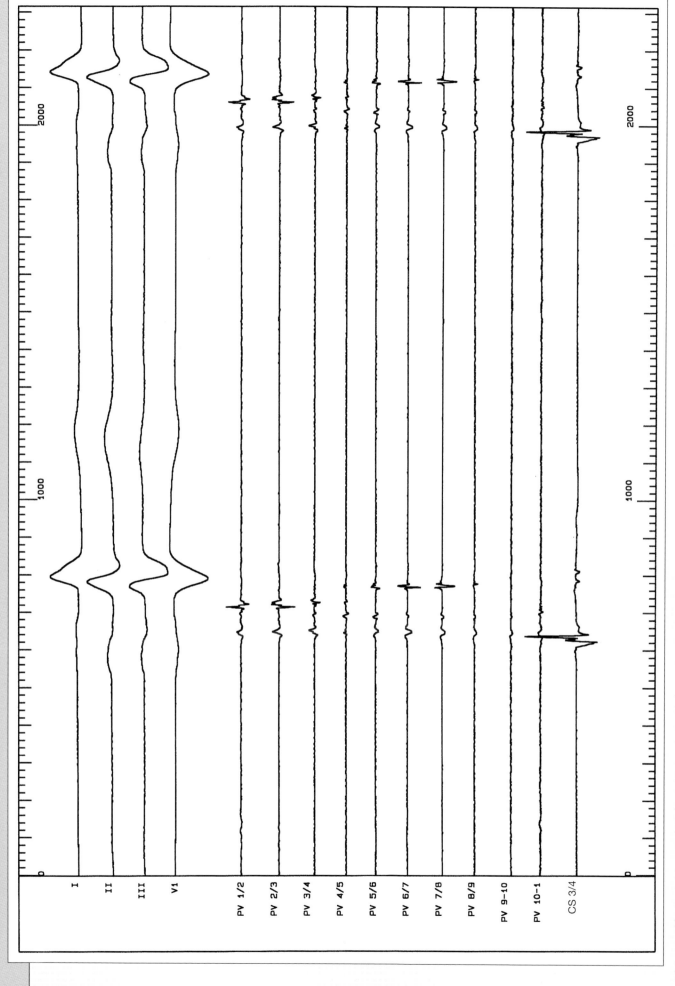

CASE 4 PART 6

- Once again, there is conduction recovery in this vein. This tracing shows not only delayed PVPs (solid line) – which can be easily distinguished from the atrial signal (dotted line) without the need for CS pacing – but also double-fractionated PVPs (double solid line), which may be seen in cases of conduction recovery and represent slow/impaired conduction.

In this case, a relatively early, low-amplitude signal is recorded at the bottom of the vein (LASSO bipoles 4/5 and 5/6). This is a common site of conduction recovery due to the presence of thicker muscular sleeves. If there is doubt about the breakthrough, CS pacing will further separate the atrial and PV signals.

Paper speed 100 mm/s

CASE 5 PART 1

- Prior to any ablation, spontaneous termination and initiation of AFIB are observed while the LASSO catheter is placed in the LSPV (the LASSO shaft is at the top of the vein).

What is the ablation target?

Paper speed 100 mm/s

III

V1

PV 1/2

PV 2/3

PV 3/4

PV 4/5

PV 5/6

PV 6/7

PV 7/8

PV 8/9

PV 9-10

PV 10-1

CS 3/4

2000

1000

31

CASE 5 PART 2

- The first part of the tracing (prior to termination) shows "organized activity" recorded during AFIB. This "organized activity" is seen in 37% of veins at baseline and probably represents less extensive PV to LA connections. Note that atrial (A) and ventricular (V) activities are quite distinct from PVPs (*).

There is a single sinus beat with fusion of the atrial and PV signals (box). Reinitiation defines the first ablation target as LASSO pole 7 at the bottom posterior segment of the vein – there is rapid repetitive firing (*) from the vein with a cascade of PV activity, commencing with polarity reversal at bipoles 6/7 and 7/8 (arrow).

Paper speed 100 mm/s

III

V1

PV 1/2

PV 2/3

PV 3/4

PV 4/5

PV 5/6

PV 6/7

PV 7/8

PV 8/9

PV 9-10

PV 10-1

CS 3/4

CASE 6 PART 1

- This tracing shows LASSO recordings from an LSPV (the LASSO shaft is at the top of the vein) after energy delivery during CS pacing.

  What is your interpretation of this recording?

  Is further ablation required?

Paper speed 100 mm/s

I

II

III

V1

PV 1/2

PV 2/3

PV 3/4

PV 4/5

PV 5/6

PV 6/7

PV 7/8

PV 8/9

PV 9–10

PV 10–1

CS 3/4

2000

1000

35

CASE 6 PART 2

- The tracing shows a dissociated PVP (∗) with polarity reversal at bipoles 1/2 and 2/3, corresponding to the top anterior part of this vein. An LA far-field signal is seen after the pacing artifact (A). Dissociation is easily confirmed by using a slower paper speed (see the next tracing). PVP dissociation is an end-point for ablation as it indicates disconnection; therefore, further energy delivery is not required.

(Paper speed 100 mm/s – turn the page for 25 mm/s.)

Paper speed 100 mm/s

I

II

III

V1

PV 1/2

PV 2/3

PV 3/4

PV 4/5

PV 5/6

PV 6/7

PV 7/8

PV 8/9

PV 9-10

PV 10-1

CS 3/4

A

A

A

*

*

1000

2000

1000

2000

0

0

37

CASE 6 PART 3

- The same tracing at 25 mm/s. This clearly shows slow, dissociated PV firing (✱).

Paper speed 25 mm/s

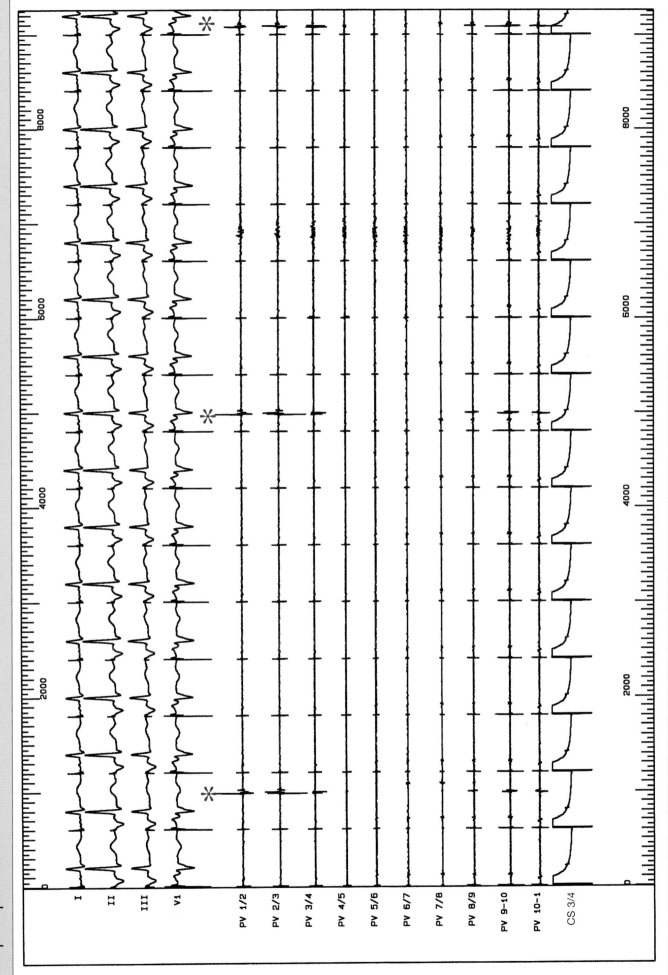

CASE 7 PART 1

- These tracings shows 12-lead ECG recordings in a patient presenting with recurrent AFIB, prior to the introduction of any catheters.

What is the likely origin of this arrhythmia?

(Note the paper speed.)

Paper speed 25 mm/s

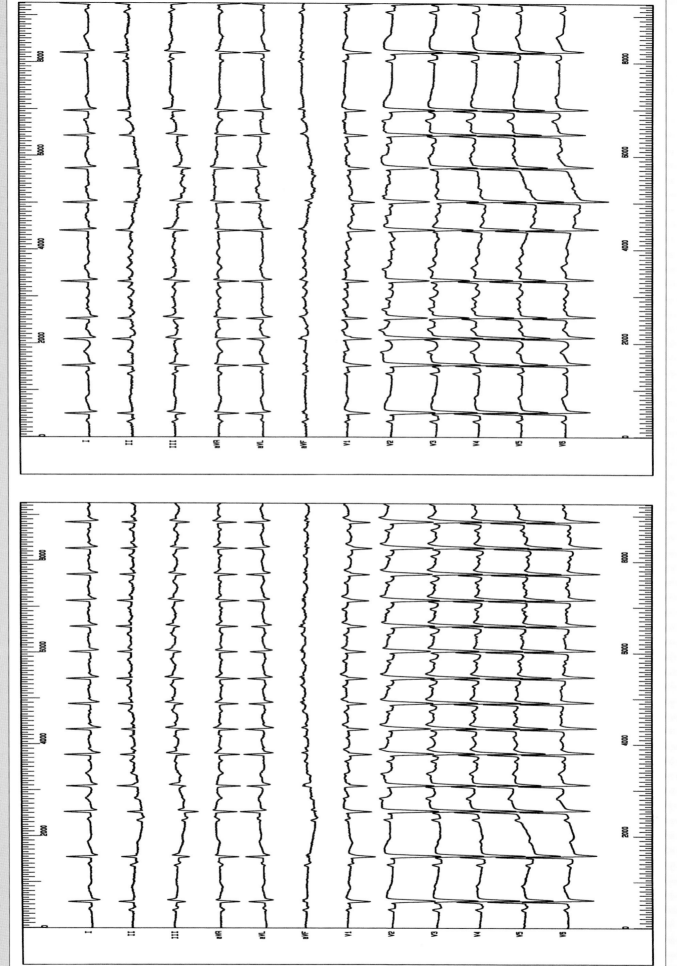

CASE 7 PART 2

- The same closely coupled atrial ectopic or "p-on-T" ectopic (✲) is responsible for tachycardia initiation. The left panel shows initiation of LA focal tachycardia, while the right panel shows initiation of AFIB followed by spontaneous termination.

  Numerous algorithms may be used to help guide ablation – one example is given on the next page.

Paper speed 25 mm/s

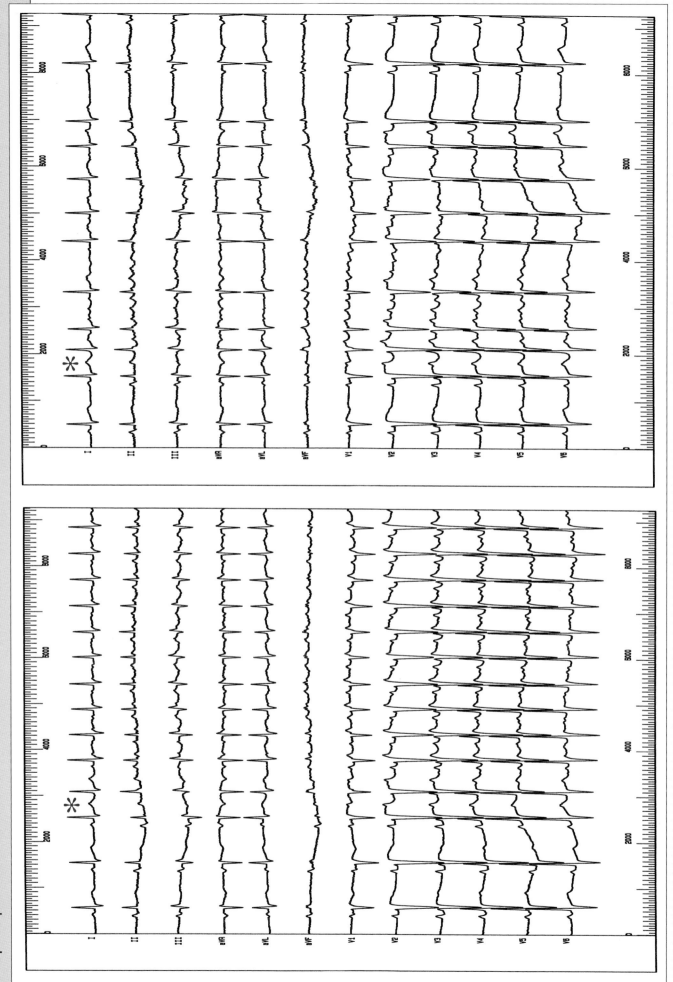

CASE 7 PART 3

- Algorithm developed by Yamane[a] for identification of the PV source of atrial ectopy. The ectopic in question probably originates from the RIPV.

P+: positive P wave.

[a]Yamane T, Shah DC, Peng JT, et al. Morphological characteristics of P waves during selective pulmonary vein pacing. J Am Coll Cardiol 2001;38:1505–10.

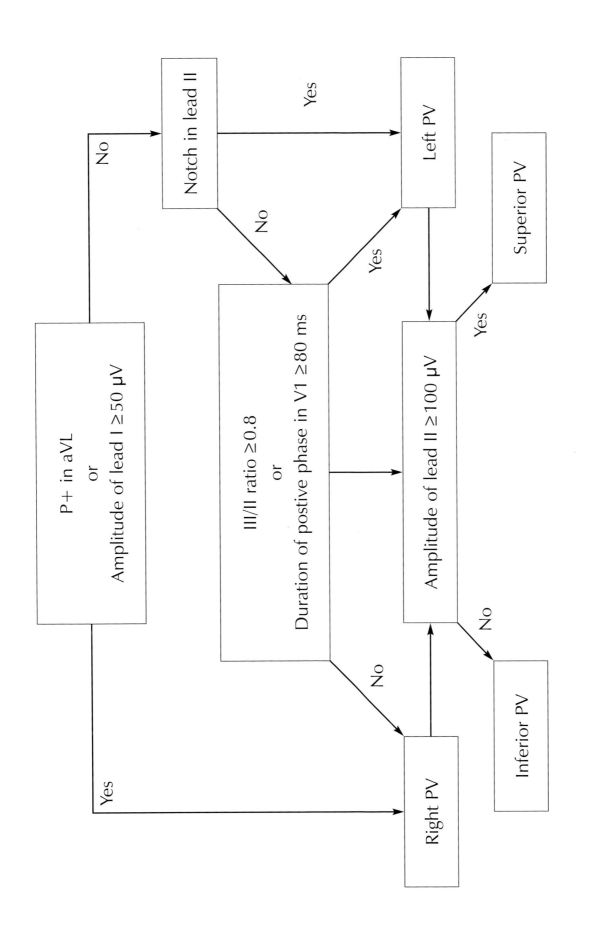

CASE 7 PART 4

- The following tracings (7.4–7.6) show mapping from various sites searching for the source of tachycardia, while tracings 7.7–7.11 are interpretations and case commentary.

- LAA mapping during clinical focal LA tachycardia.

Paper speed 100 mm/s

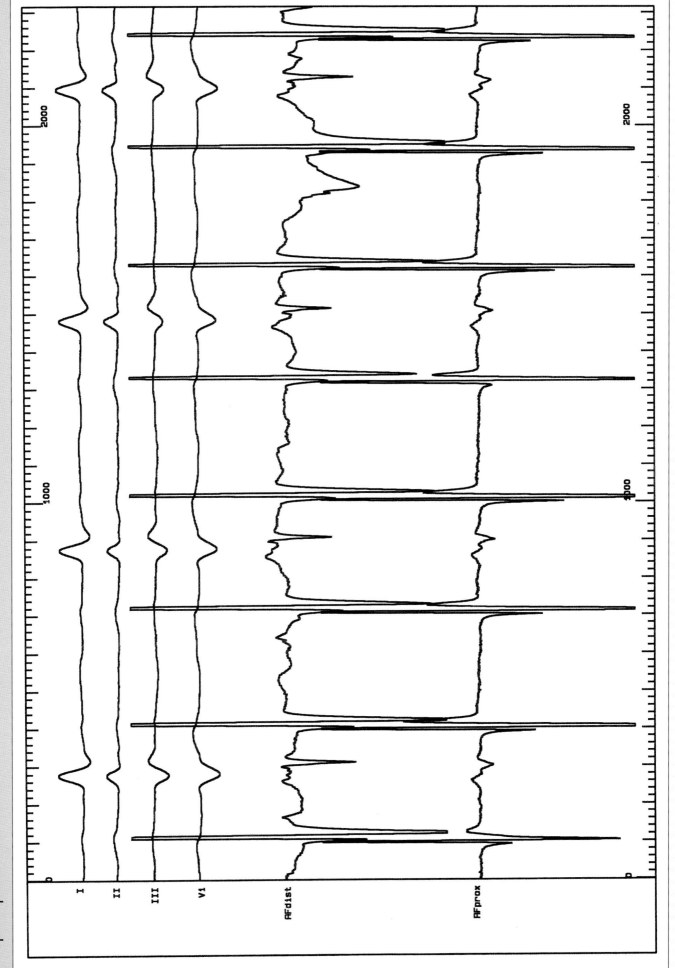

CASE 7 PART 5

- Septal LA mapping during clinical focal LA tachycardia.

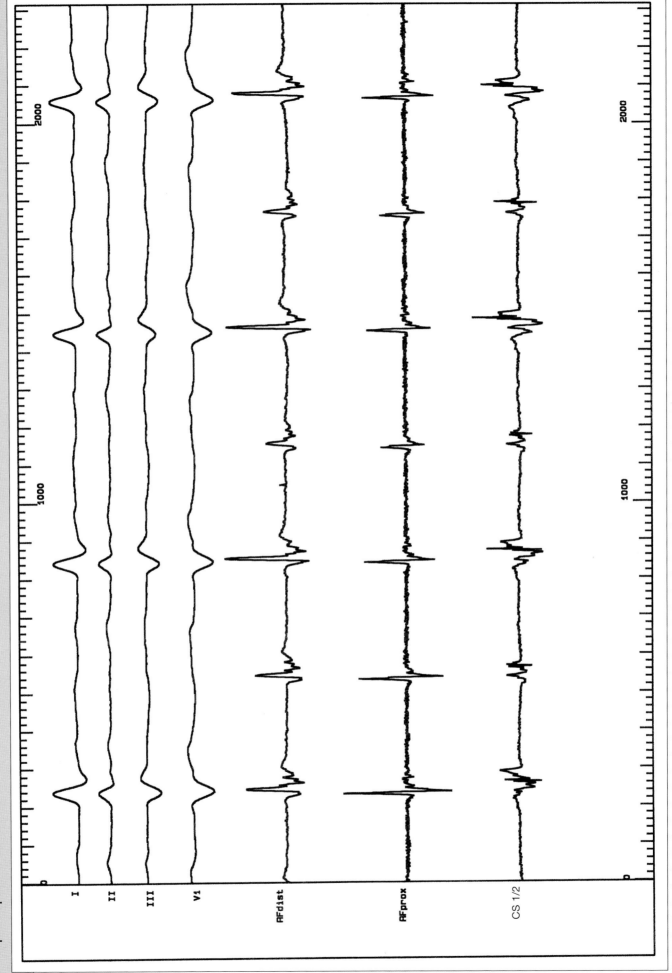

CASE 7 PART 6

- Mapping the bottom part of the RIPV ostium during clinical LA tachycardia.

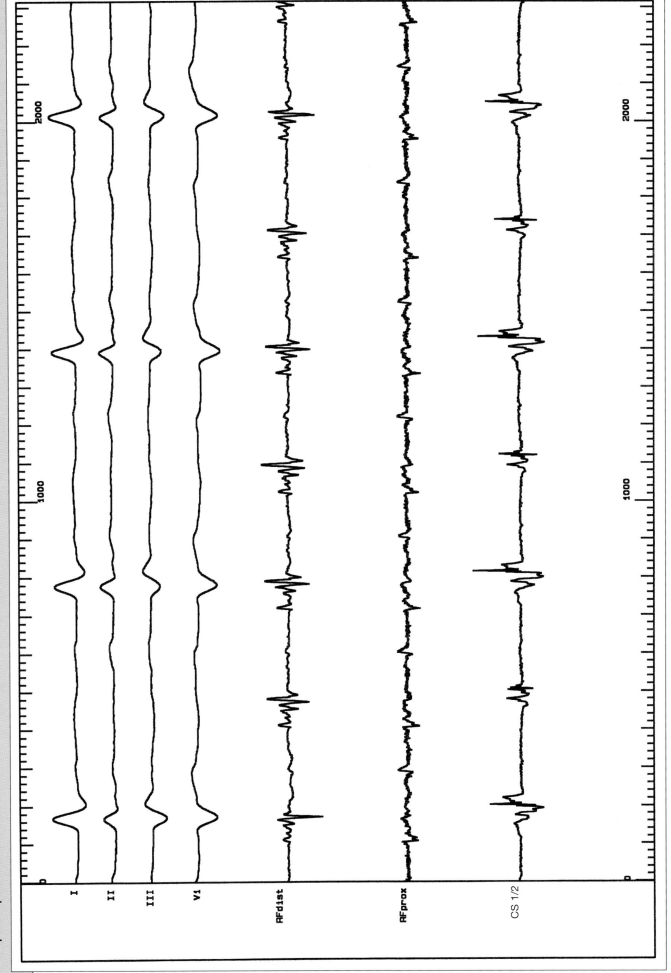

Paper speed 100 mm/s

CASE 7 PART 7

- The LAA recording is late (dotted line) compared with the surface P wave during tachycardia – this is clearly not the ablation target.

Paper speed 100 mm/s

CASE 7 PART 8

- The septal LA site is early (dotted line) with respect to the surface P wave during tachycardia.

Paper speed 100 mm/s

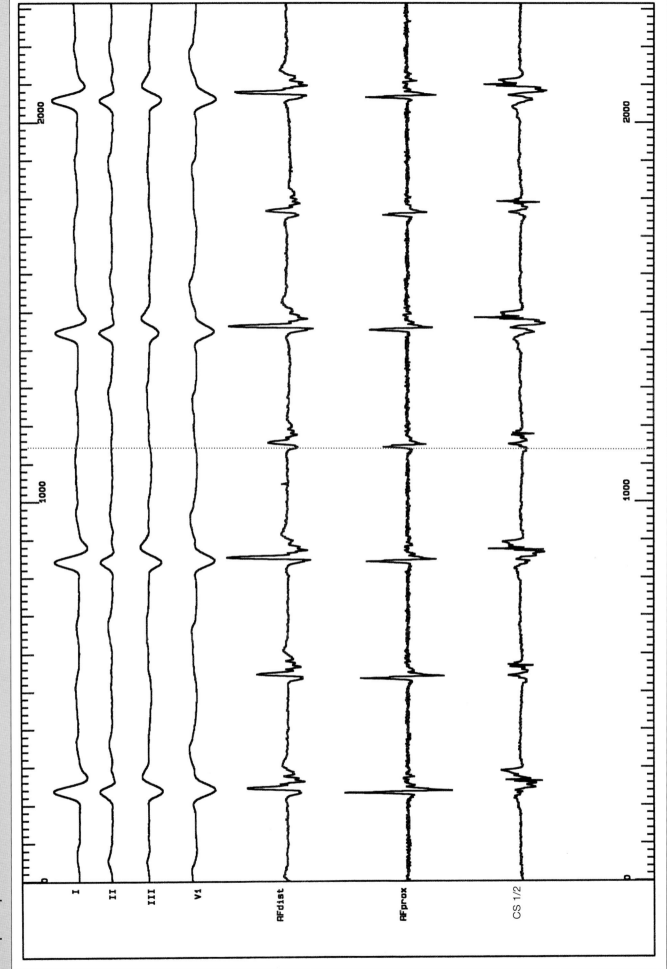

- Early fractionated activity (✽) compared with the atrial signal (A) in the CS and the surface P wave indicates that the ablation target is at the ostium of the RIPV. Ostial foci are a frequent cause of AFIB recurrence.

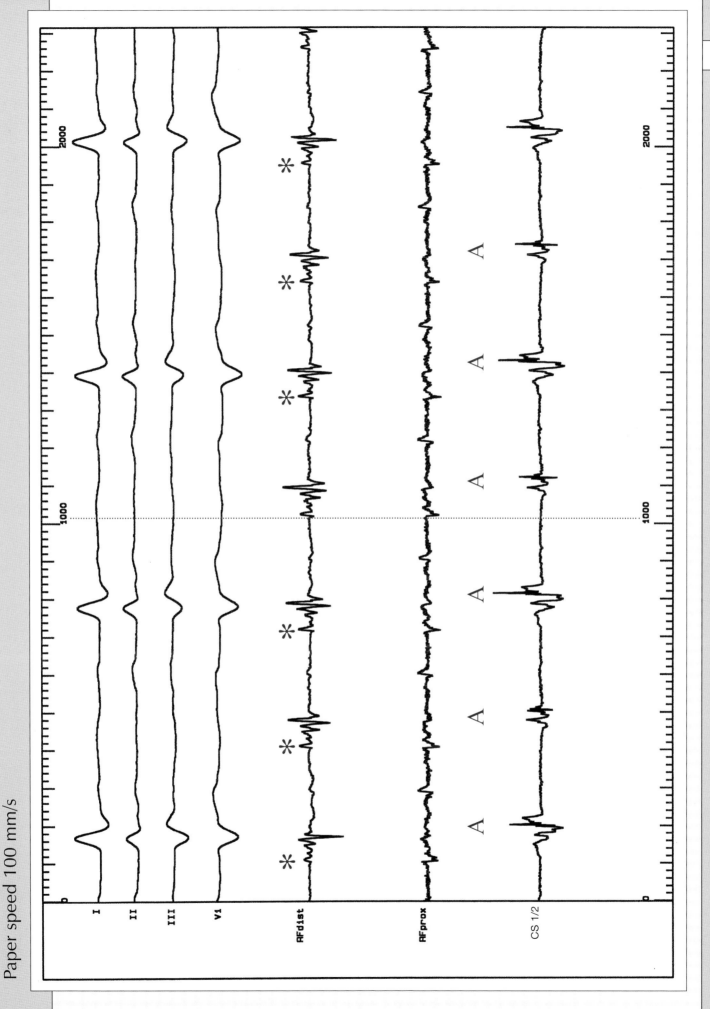

Paper speed 100 mm/s

- In the same patient, there was early (within 20 seconds) termination of focal arrhythmia during ablation at the bottom part of the RIPV ostium. The end-point for ablation of non-PV ectopy is less clear than for PV disconnection. It is important to observe the rhythm for some time after ablation to check for recurrence of clinical ectopy.

Paper speed 50 mm/s

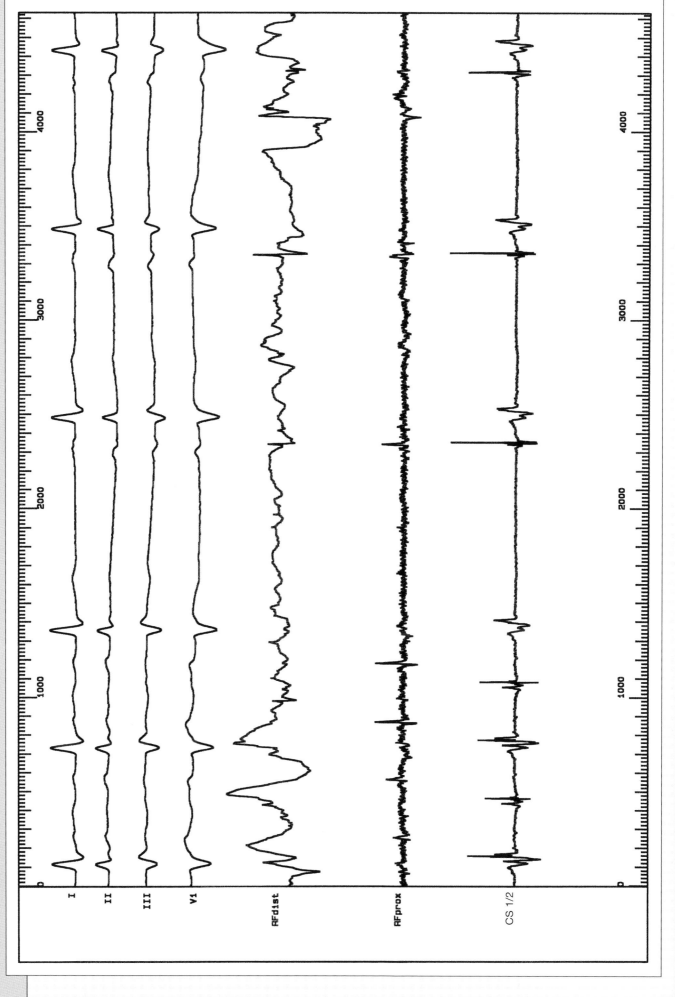

CASE 7 PART 11

- This postablation tracing shows the disappearance of ostial activity on the mapping catheter.

Paper speed 100 mm/s

I

II

III

V1

RFdist

RFprox

CS 1/2

2000

1000

CASE 8 PART 1

- This is a LASSO tracing from the LIPV during AFIB (the LASSO shaft is at the top of the vein).

  What is the ablation target?

Paper speed 100 mm/s

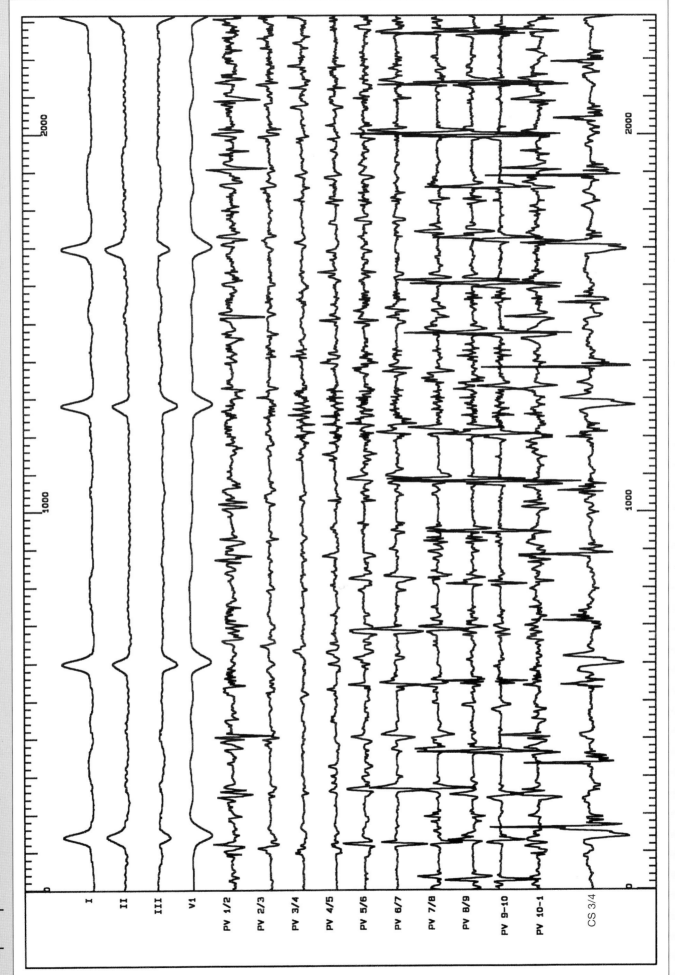

CASE 8 PART 2

- The PV activity is completely disorganized, so ablation is commenced anatomically, initially targeting the top and bottom of the vein.

Paper speed 100 mm/s

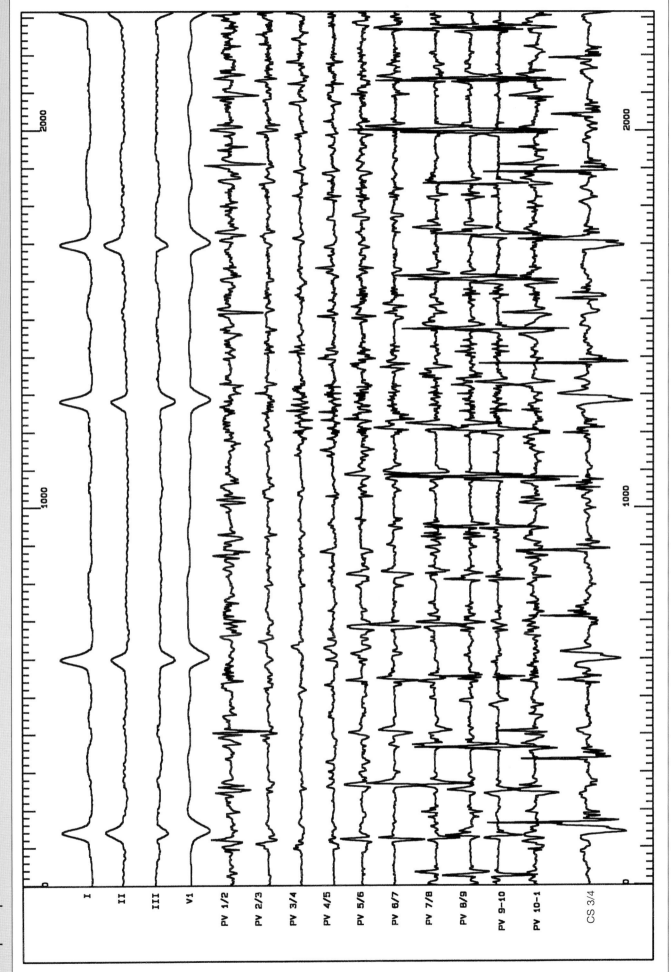

CASE 8 PART 3

- After initial anatomical ablation of the bottom of this PV, the following tracing is recorded.

  What is your interpretation?

Paper speed 100 mm/s

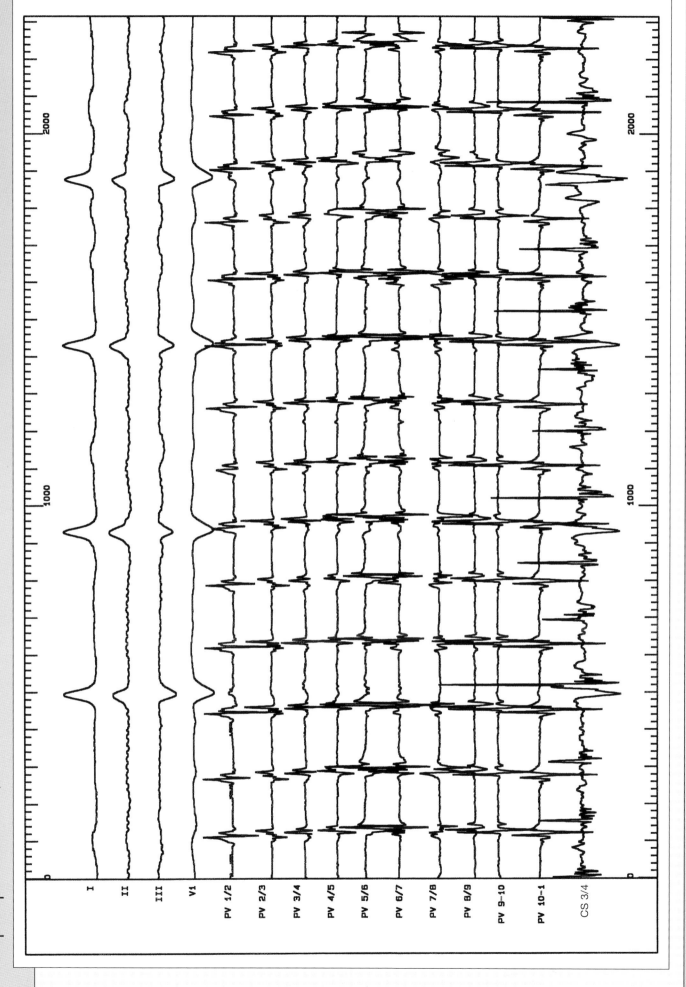

CASE 8 PART 4

- In 63% of veins, PV activity is disorganized during AFIB at baseline. In 75% of these veins, activity becomes organized following some change to the initial anatomical energy delivery. In this case, PV activation has become organized (✱) during AFIB, with the earliest activity at LASSO bipoles 1/2 and 10–1. This corresponds to the top of the vein, which would be the next ablation target.

Paper speed 100 mm/s

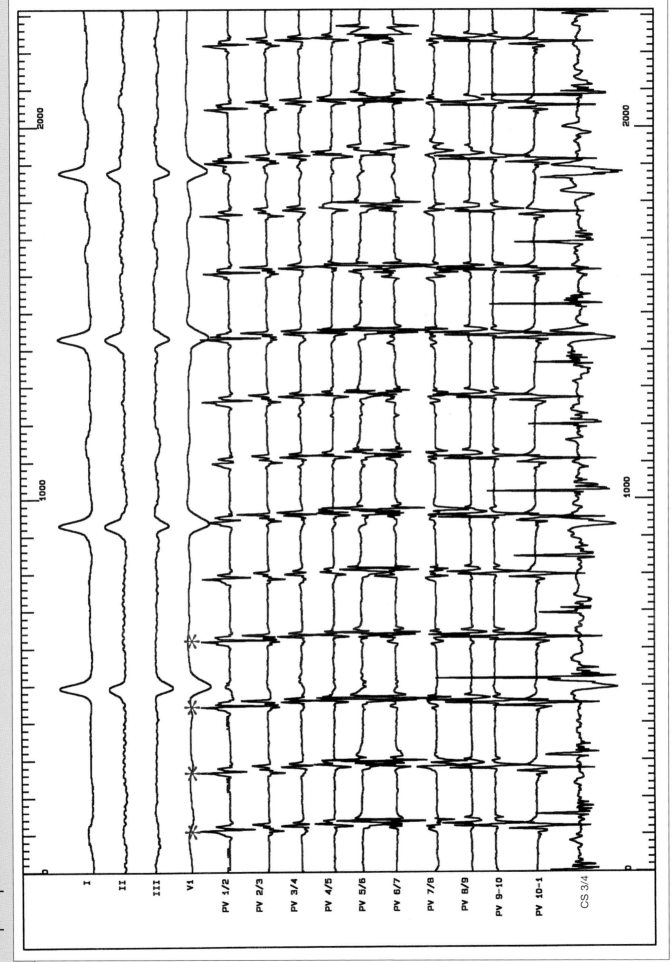

CASE 8 PART 5

- The following tracing is recorded during ablation targeting the top of the same vein (note the thermal artifact on bipoles 1/2 and 10–1).

  What is your interpretation?

Paper speed 100 mm/s

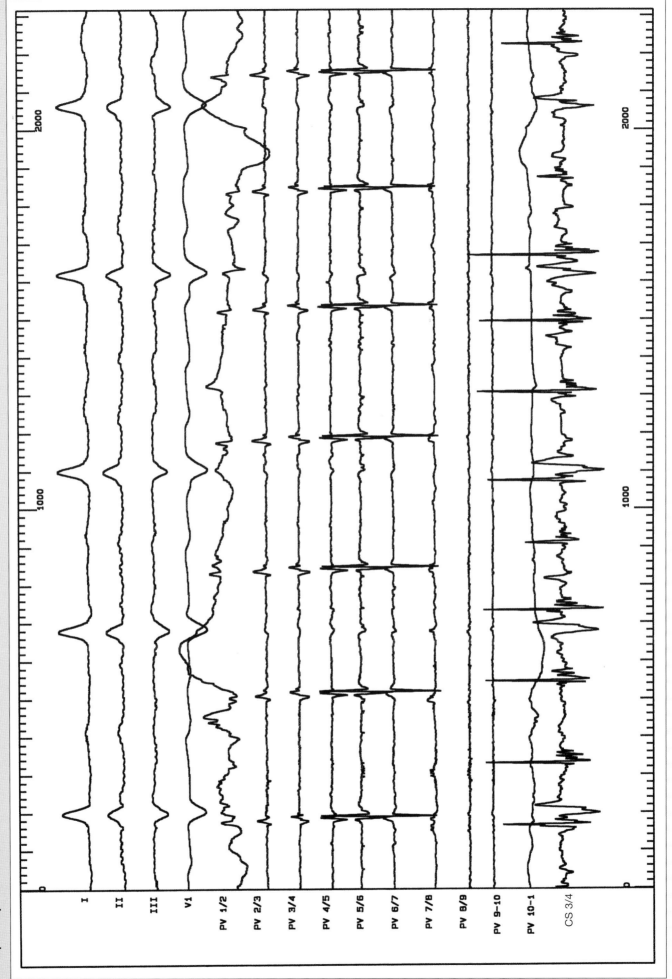

I

II

III

V1

PV 1/2

PV 2/3

PV 3/4

PV 4/5

PV 5/6

PV 6/7

PV 7/8

PV 8/9

PV 9-10

PV 10-1

CS 3/4

2000

1000

2000

1000

CASE 8 PART 6

- There is now high-grade conduction block (approximately 2:1 in comparison with the CS recording) during ongoing AFIB; this often precedes disconnection. Note the thermal artifact on bipoles 1/2 and 10–1 as RF delivery at the top of the vein is ongoing.

Paper speed 100 mm/s

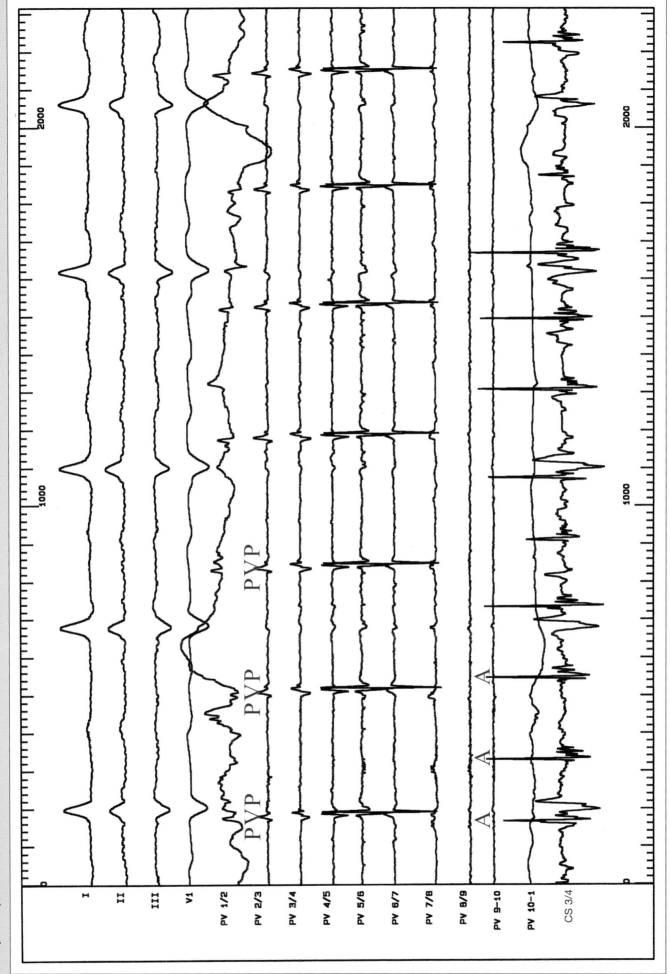

73

CASE 8 PART 7

- This tracing was recorded following RF delivery in the same vein.

What is your interpretation?

Paper speed 100 mm/s

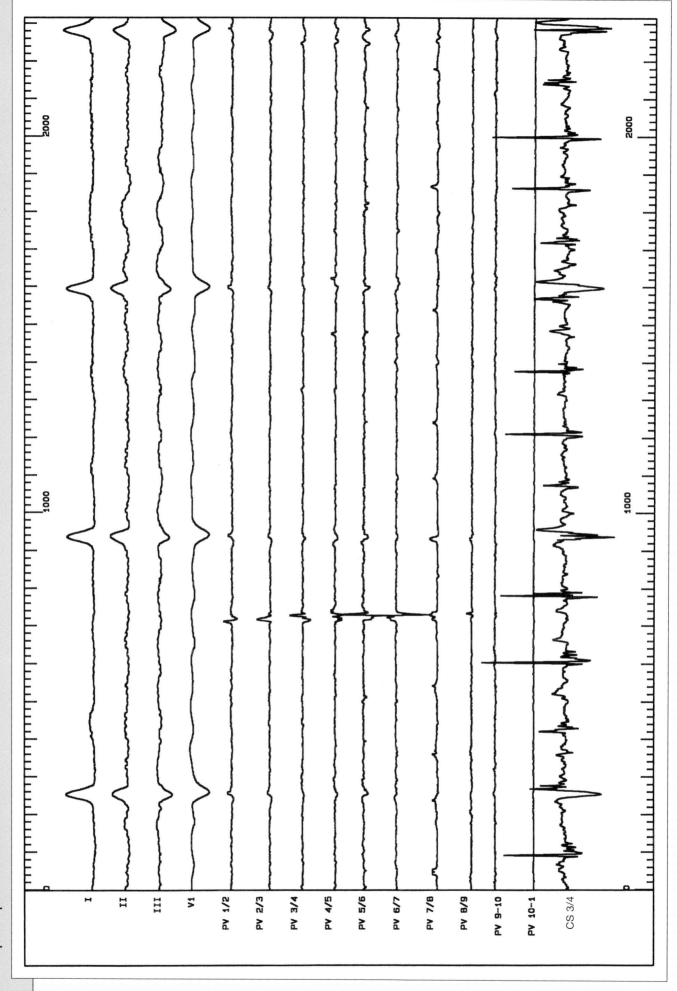

CASE 8 PART 8

- There is now PV dissociation during ongoing AFIB, with a complete sequence of PVPs recorded within the vein (✱). Atrial (A) and ventricular (V) far-field signals can also be seen.

Paper speed 100 mm/s

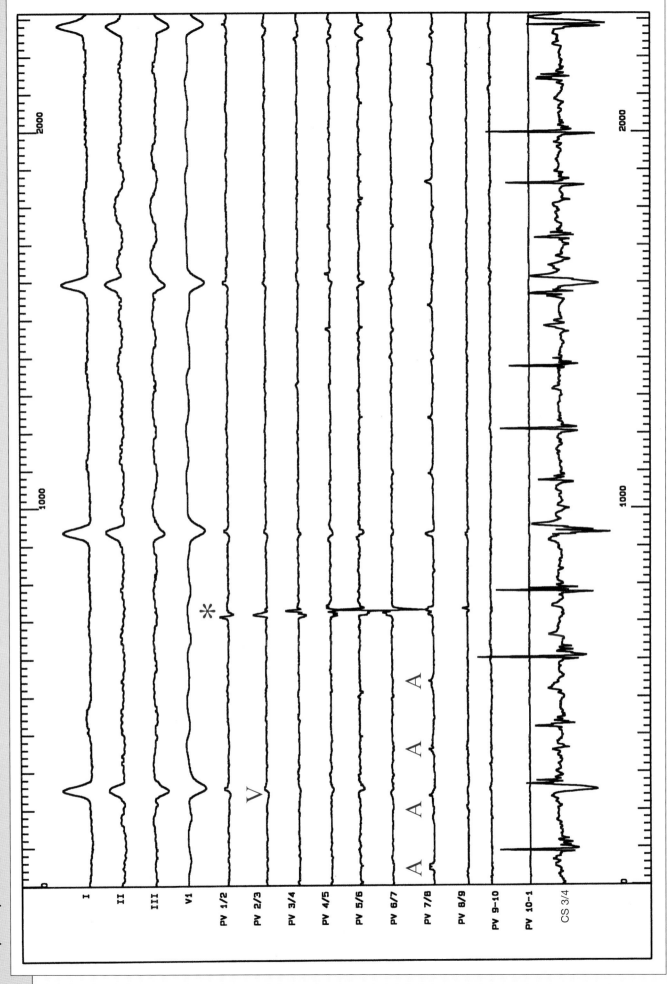

CASE 9 PART 1

- This tracing was obtained during ongoing ablation at the bottom posterior part of an LIPV (the LASSO shaft is at the top of the vein).

  What is your interpretation?

  Note: distal CS pacing.

Paper speed 100 mm/s

I
II
III
V1

PV 1/2
PV 2/3
PV 3/4
PV 4/5
PV 5/6
PV 6/7
PV 7/8
PV 8/9
PV 9-10
PV 10-1

2000

1000

2000

1000

79

CASE 9 PART 2

- There is partial disconnection during ablation, with the loss of PVP (✱) from LASSO bipoles 5/6–8/9. Note polarity reversal at LASSO bipoles 7/8 and 8/9 (arrow). Conduction is already slow at this site as a result of ablation, explaining why PVPs at this site are no longer the earliest.

Paper speed 100 mm/s

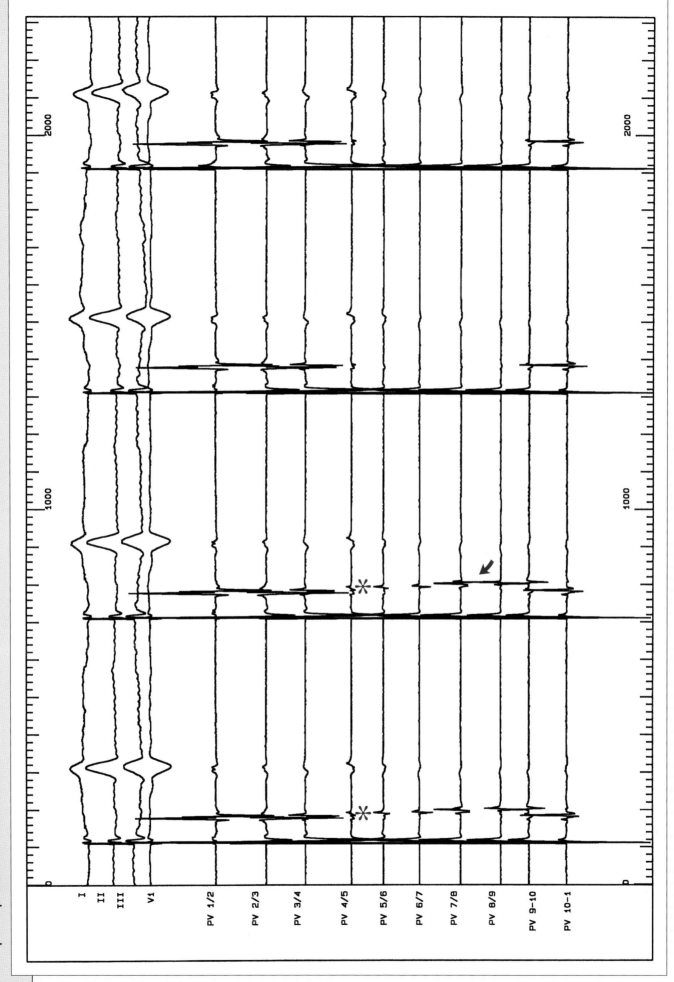

- What is the next ablation target?

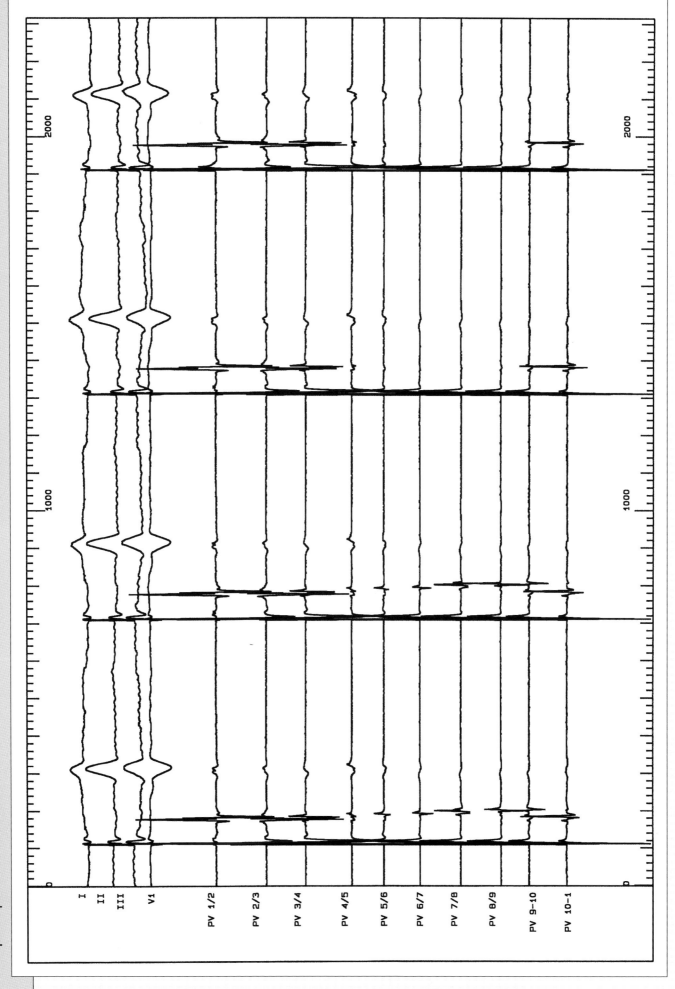

Paper speed 100 mm/s

CASE 9 PART 4

- Before moving to the next ablation target, it is important to adequately ablate the current site with a minimum of 60 seconds ablation after local disappearance of PVPs. The next ablation target is LASSO bipole 2/3 at the top anterior part of this vein – this is because the earliest PVP (*) is there, together with polarity reversal (arrow).

Paper speed 100 mm/s

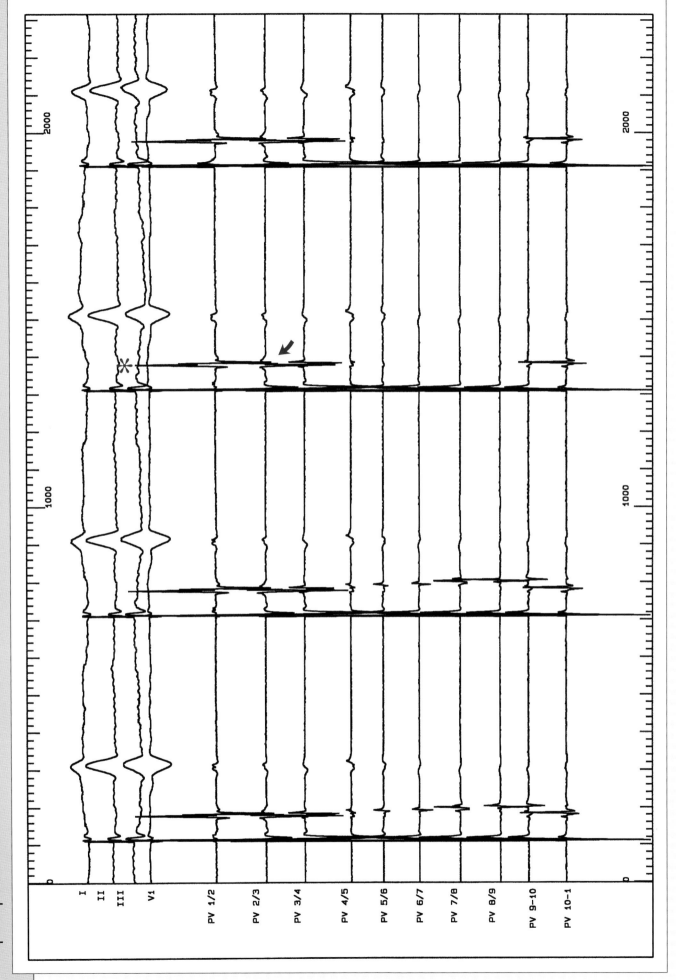

CASE 9 PART 5

- During ablation targeting LASSO pole 2 in the same LSPV, the following tracing was recorded.

What is your interpretation?

Paper speed 100 mm/s

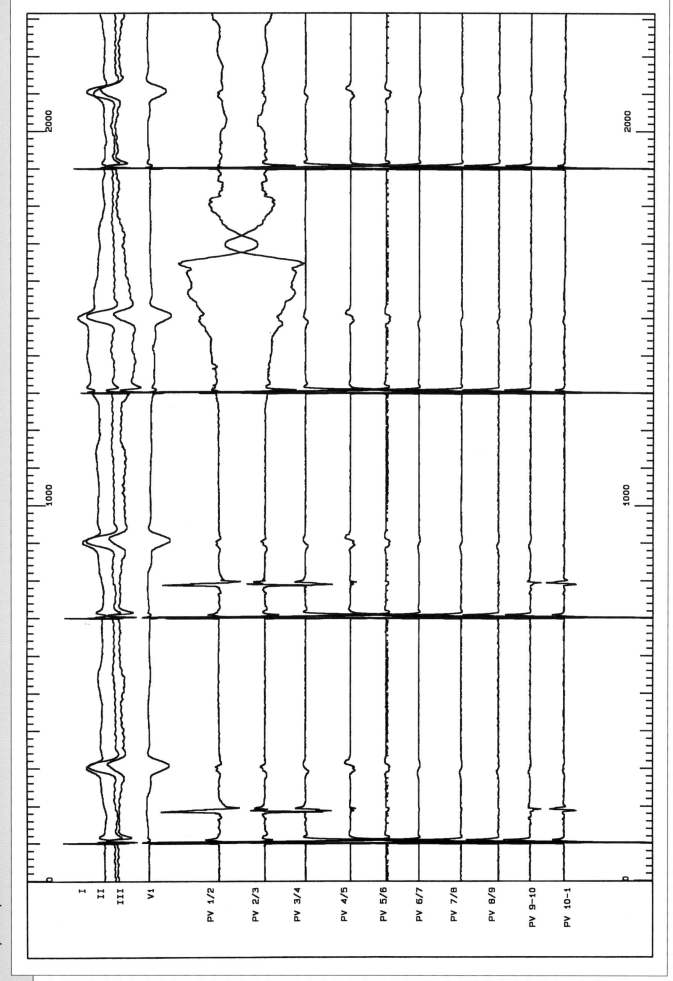

I
II
III
V1
PV 1/2
PV 2/3
PV 3/4
PV 4/5
PV 5/6
PV 6/7
PV 7/8
PV 8/9
PV 9-10
PV 10-1

2000

1000

2000

1000

- The vein has been completely disconnected with loss of all PVPs (✳). Note the thermal artifact at bipoles 1/2 and 2/3 (arrow).

Paper speed 100 mm/s

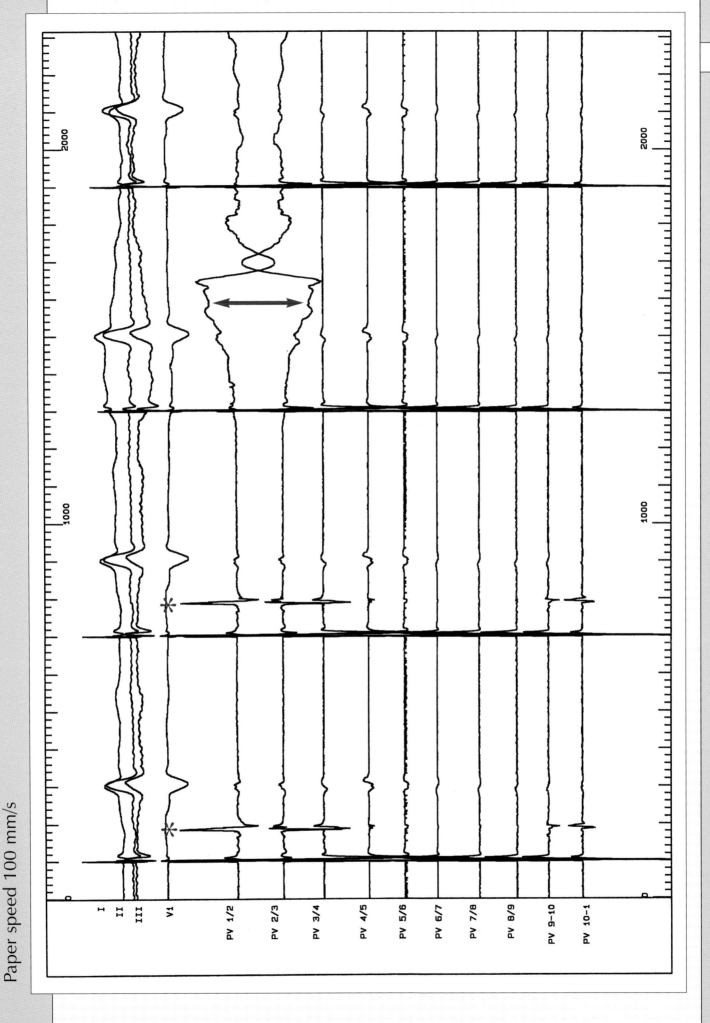

CASE 10 PART 1

- This tracing is from an RSPV during AFIB (the LASSO shaft is at the top of the vein). There is ongoing ablation at LASSO pole 5.

Is the venous conduction pattern organized or disorganized?

Paper speed 100 mm/s

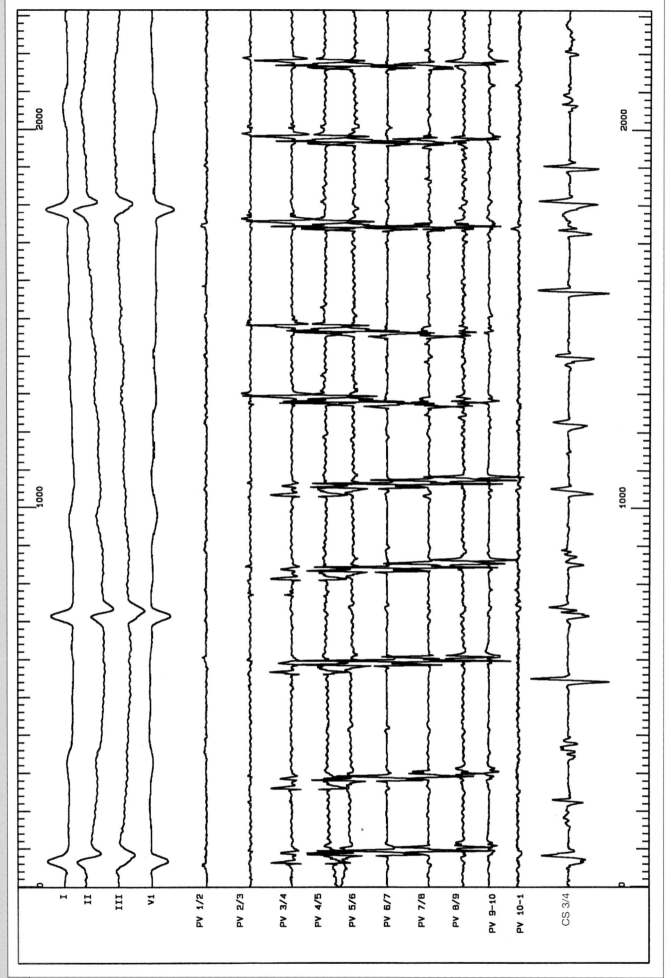

- The venous pattern is organized during AFIB, with two distinct patterns visible (✳ and ★). The first breakthrough has been abolished by ablation at the bottom of the vein and there has been a change in activation. The arrows represent the two breakthroughs visible on this tracing.

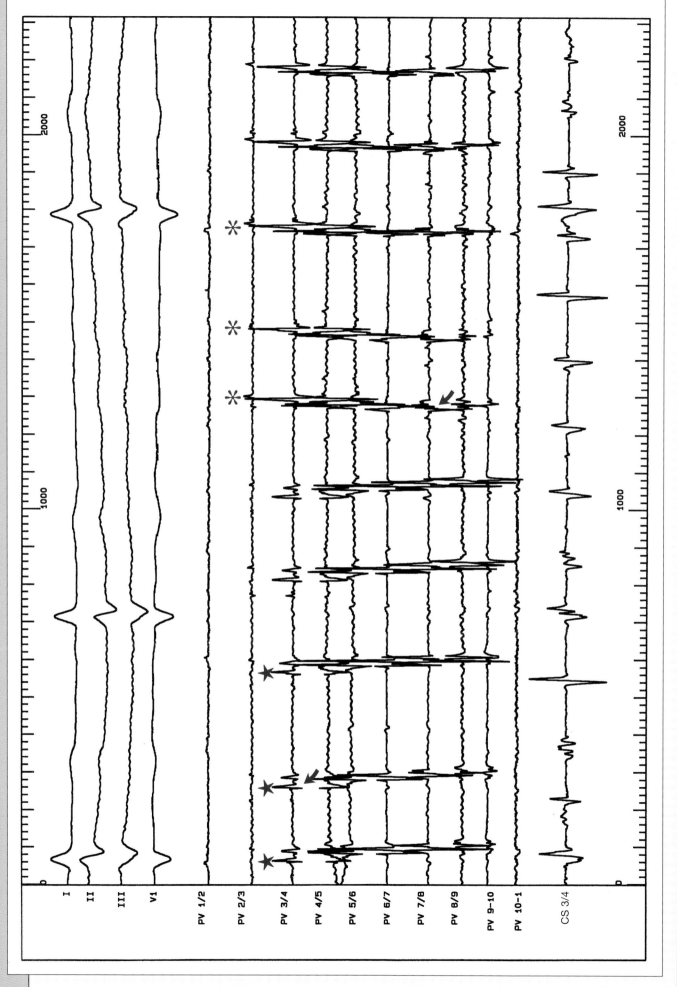

Paper speed 100 mm/s

I

II

III

V1

PV 1/2

PV 2/3

PV 3/4

PV 4/5

PV 5/6

PV 6/7

PV 7/8

PV 8/9

PV 9-10

PV 10-1

CS 3/4

CASE 11 PART 1

- The following tracing is recorded during ablation of the posterior wall of the LSPV.

What is your interpretation?

Paper speed 12.5 mm/s

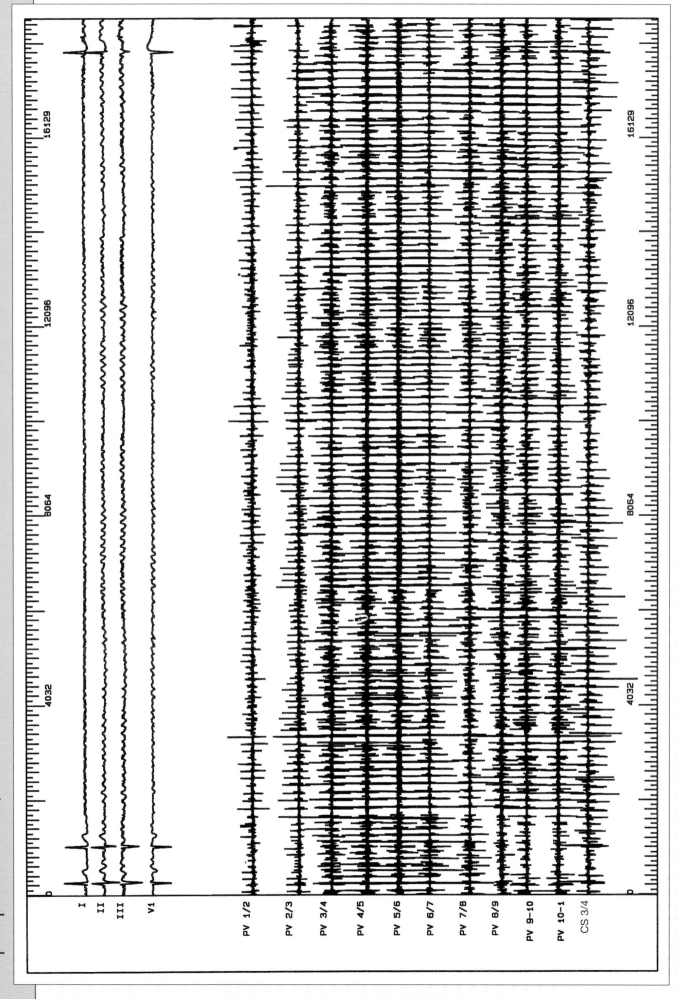

CASE 11 PART 2

- This tracing shows a long ventricular pause during ablation (dotted line). This is presumably a vagally mediated phenomenon. It most frequently occurs during ablation of the posterior wall of the left veins, which is often painful for the patient. This can easily be overlooked if the screen speed is 100 mm/s.

Paper speed 12.5 mm/s

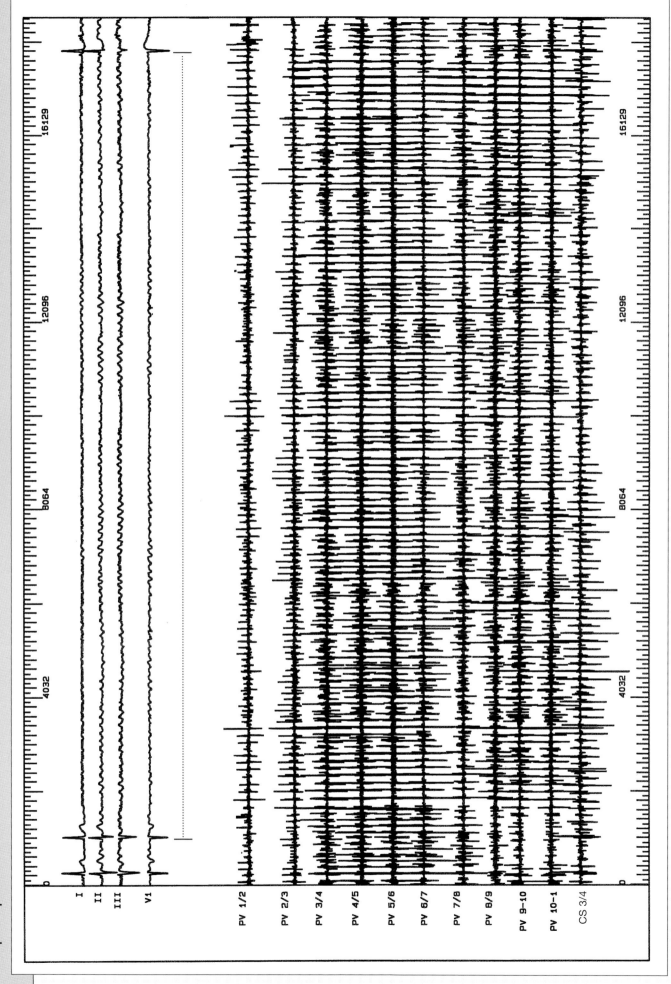

CASE 12 PART 1

- This tracing is from an LSPV during sinus rhythm prior to ablation (the LASSO shaft is at the bottom posterior part of the vein).

What is the ablation target?

Paper speed 100 mm/s

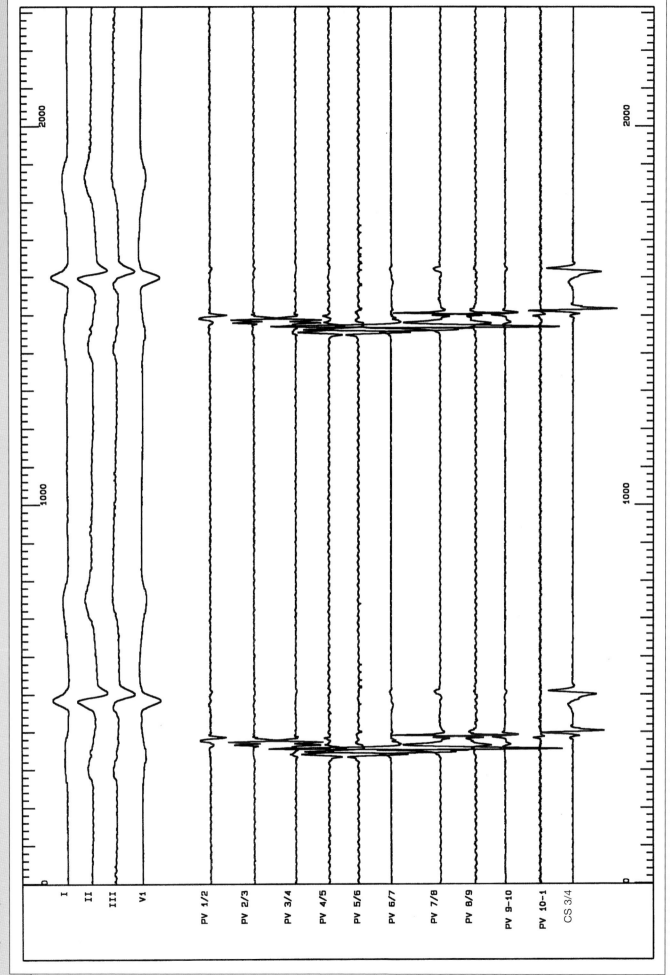

CASE 12 PART 2

- The ablation target is unclear because the LA far-field and PVP signals are fused during sinus rhythm. Delayed PVP on LASSO bipoles 7/8 (arrow) should be suspected. To confirm this, it is crucial to pace the distal CS or LA appendage in order to clearly see the PVPs.

Paper speed 100 mm/s

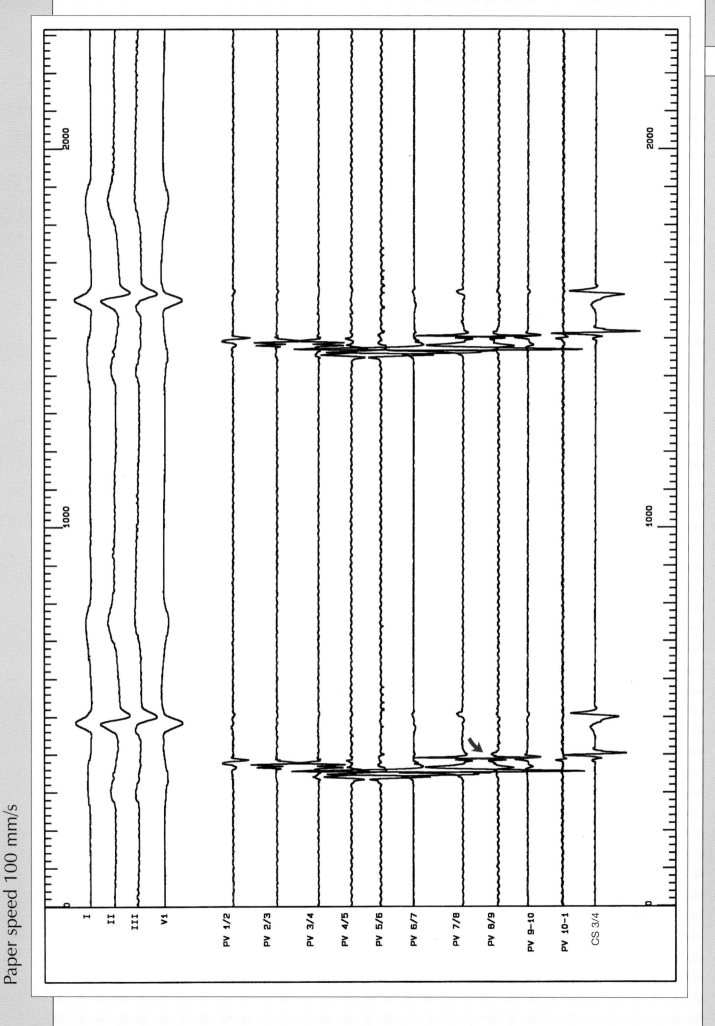

2000

1000

2000

1000

I

II

III

V1

PV 1/2

PV 2/3

PV 3/4

PV 4/5

PV 5/6

PV 6/7

PV 7/8

PV 8/9

PV 9-10

PV 10-1

CS 3/4

- This tracing shows CS pacing in the same vein (the LASSO shaft is at the bottom posterior part of the vein).

  Where is the ablation target?

Paper speed 100 mm/s

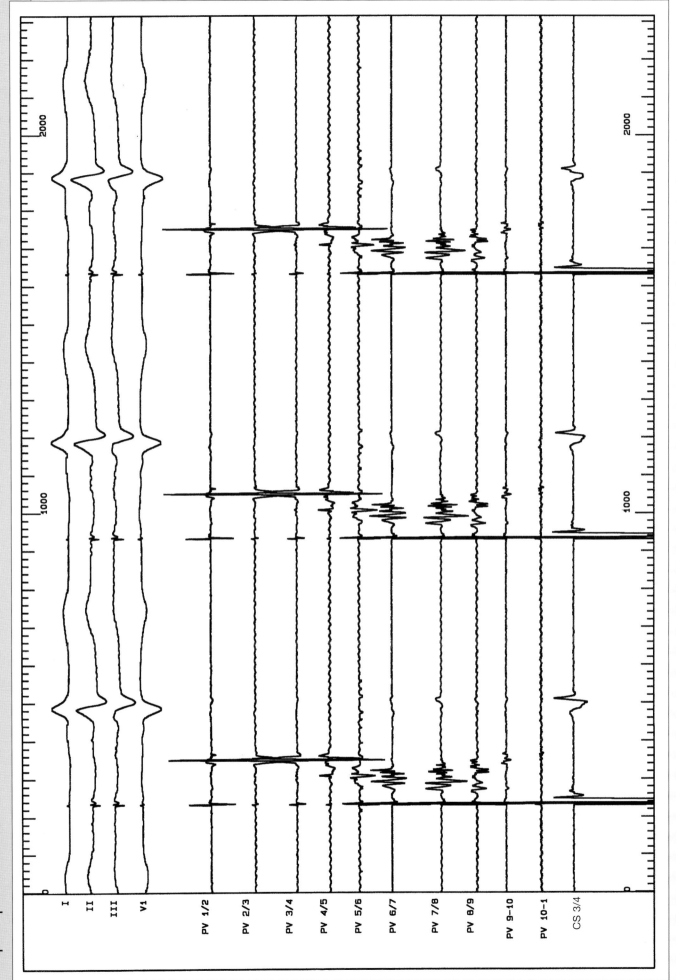

CASE 12 PART 4

- Delayed spike potential is clearly visible on bipoles 1/2–4/5, with the typical appearance of a PVP (∗). There is a fractionated signal on LASSO bipoles 6/7–8/9, corresponding to the posterior wall of this vein. This fractionated signal represents fusion of the LAA far-field signal (A) with the earliest PVP (arrow) because the LASSO is positioned very near the ostium. The initial ablation target would be pole 7.

Paper speed 100 mm/s

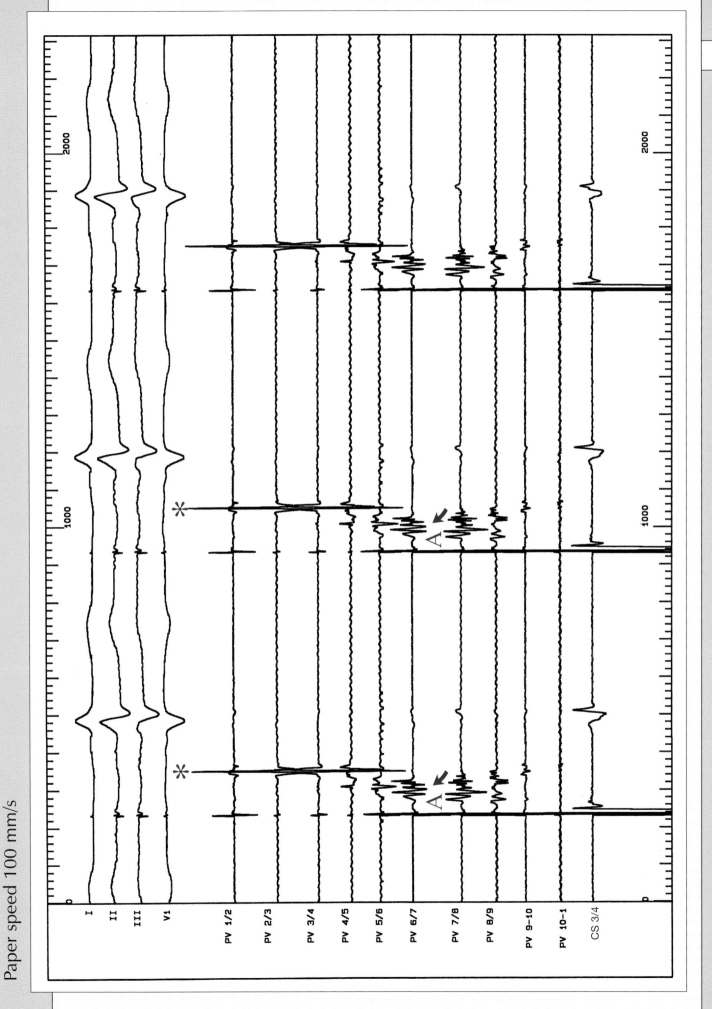

I

II

III

V1

PV 1/2

PV 2/3

PV 3/4

PV 4/5

PV 5/6

PV 6/7

PV 7/8

PV 8/9

PV 9-10

PV 10-1

CS 3/4

CASE 12 PART 5

- During energy delivery at LASSO pole 5 in the same vein, the following tracing is recorded.

  What is your interpretation?

Paper speed 100 mm/s

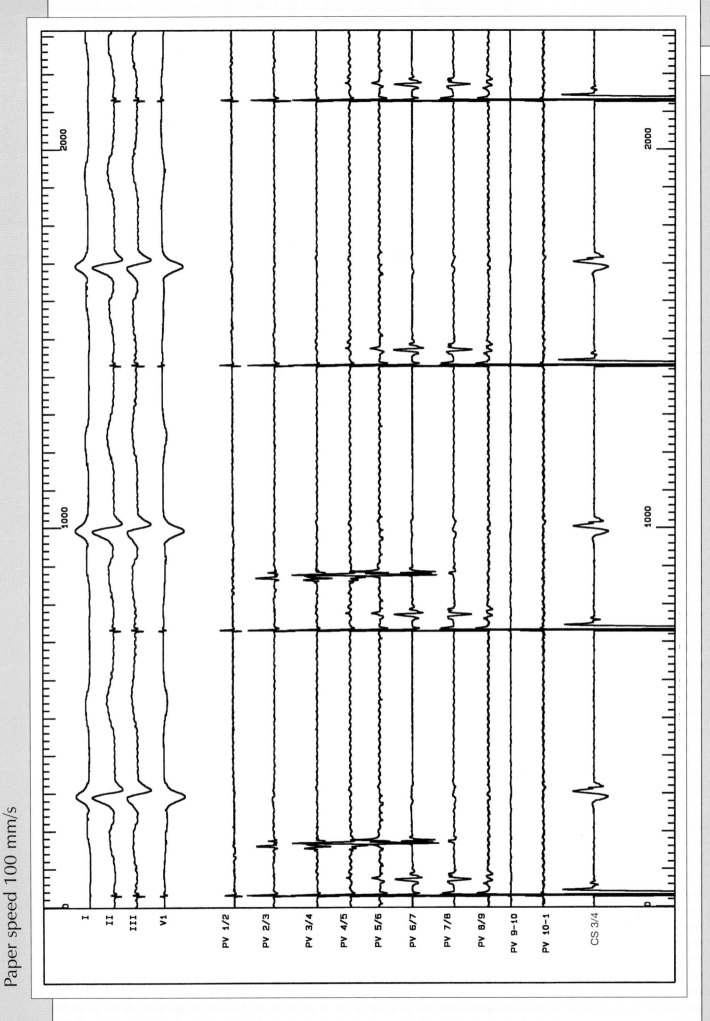

CASE 12 PART 6

- Following initial ablation, the atrial far-field signal (A) is now clearly distinct from the PVPs (✱). The PVPs are also delayed and disappear during energy delivery. Energy delivery should be continued for at least 60 seconds more at this site to ensure adequate ablation and reduce the risk of recovery.

Paper speed 100 mm/s

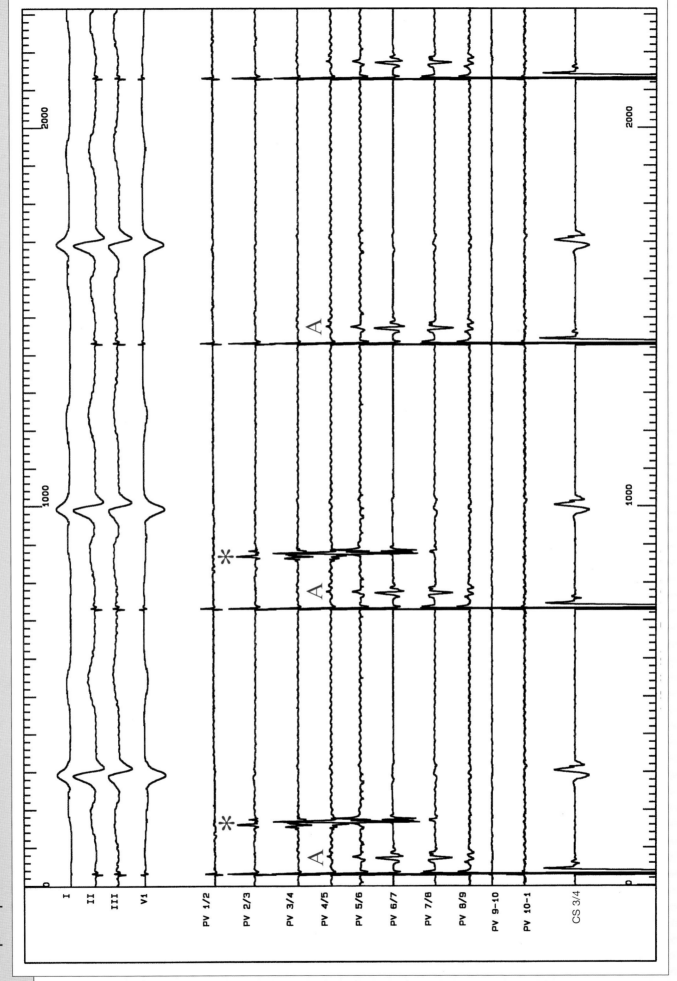

CASE 13 PART 1

- This tracing is from an RSPV prior to ablation (the LASSO shaft is at the top of the vein).

  What is your interpretation?

Paper speed 100 mm/s

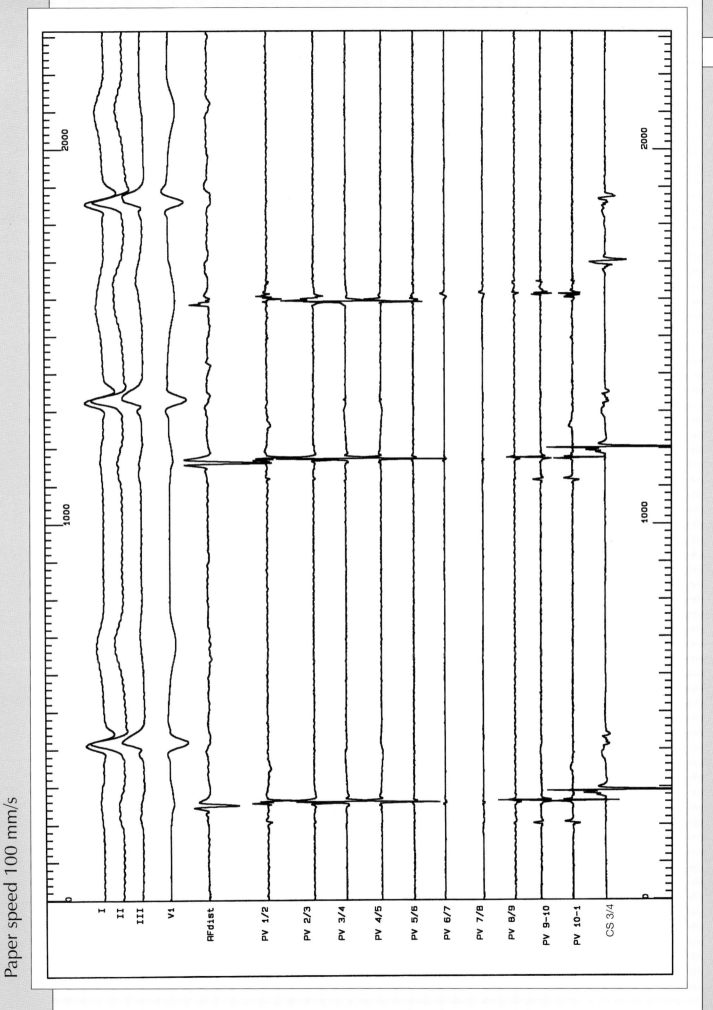

CASE 13 PART 2

- The LASSO is relatively deep within the PV, explaining the delay between the atrial far-field signal (A) and the PVP. This also demonstrates activation reversal, with a local ectopic (∗) from the PV followed by atrial signals. Note that the ablation catheter signal is early and represents a good ablation target (dotted line).

Paper speed 100 mm/s

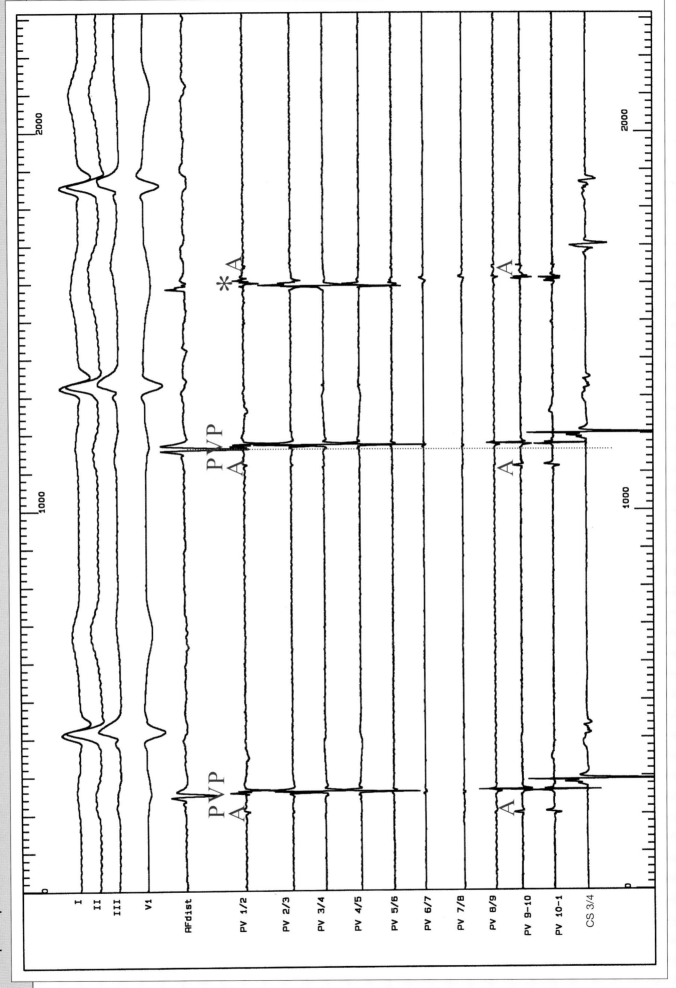

- Which vein/ostium is likely to be responsible for this initiation of AFIB?

Paper speed 25 mm/s

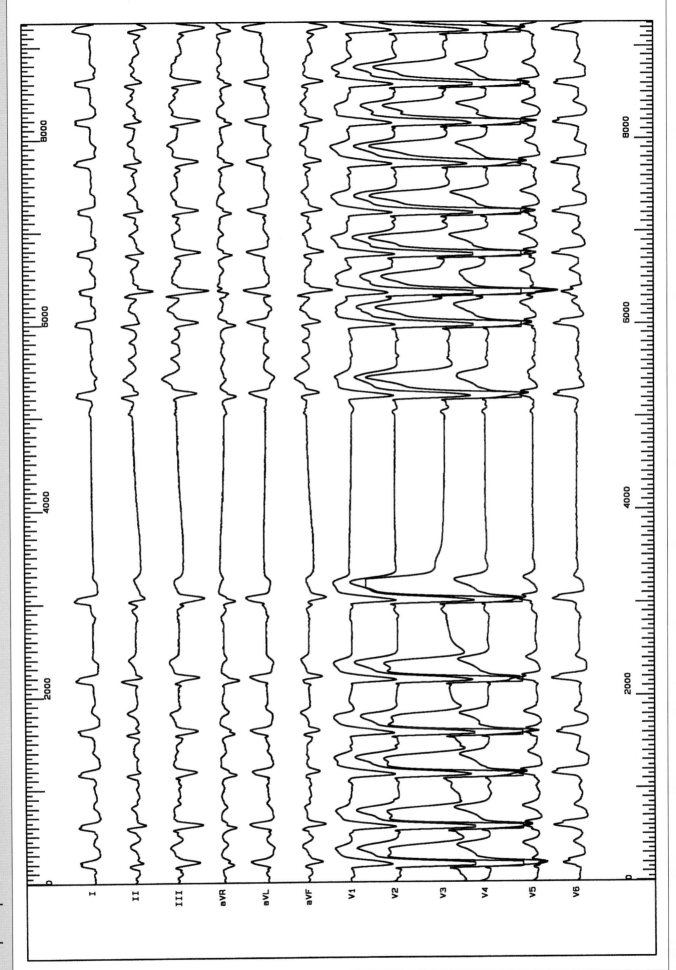

CASE 13 PART 4

- The ectopic P wave is negative in lead I, positive in leads II and III, and negative in aVL. Using the algorithm on page 45, it is likely to be from the LSPV.

Paper speed 25 mm/s

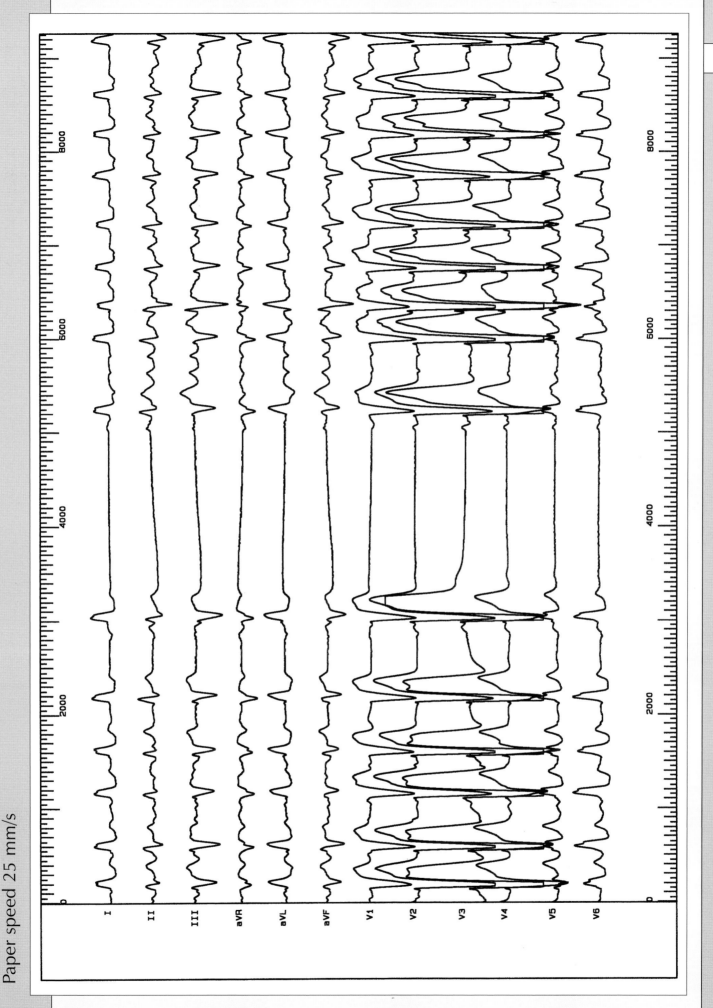

CASE 14 PART 1

- This recording is from an LIPV prior to any ablation during CS pacing.

  What is the ablation target?

Paper speed 100 mm/s

I
II
III
V1

RFdist

PV 1/2
PV 2/3
PV 3/4
PV 4/5
PV 5/6
PV 6/7
PV 7/8
PV 8/9
PV 9-10
PV 10-1

CS 3/4

1000   2000

119

- All of the PVPs line up without any apparent "cascade" (dotted line). There appears to be polarity reversal around LASSO pole 9 (arrow), which could be confirmed by reducing the size of the PV signals so that they do not overlap. Polarity reversal can be used to select an ablation target when there is no obvious "cascade".

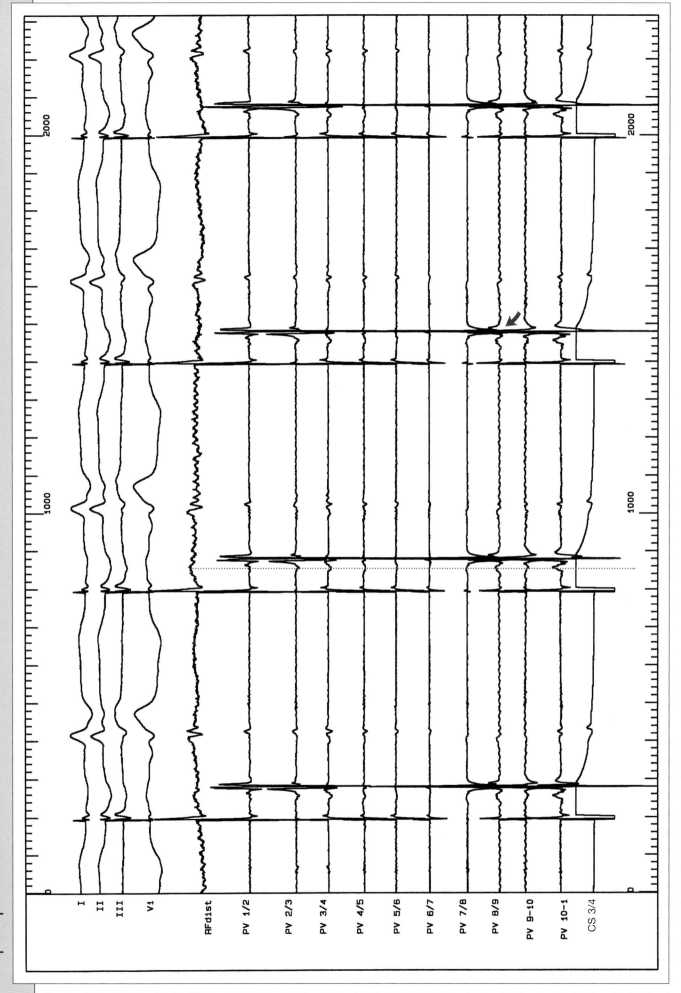

Paper speed 100 mm/s

- This tracing is from an RSPV (the LASSO shaft is at the top of the vein).

  What is your interpretation of the second and third beats?

Paper speed 100 mm/s

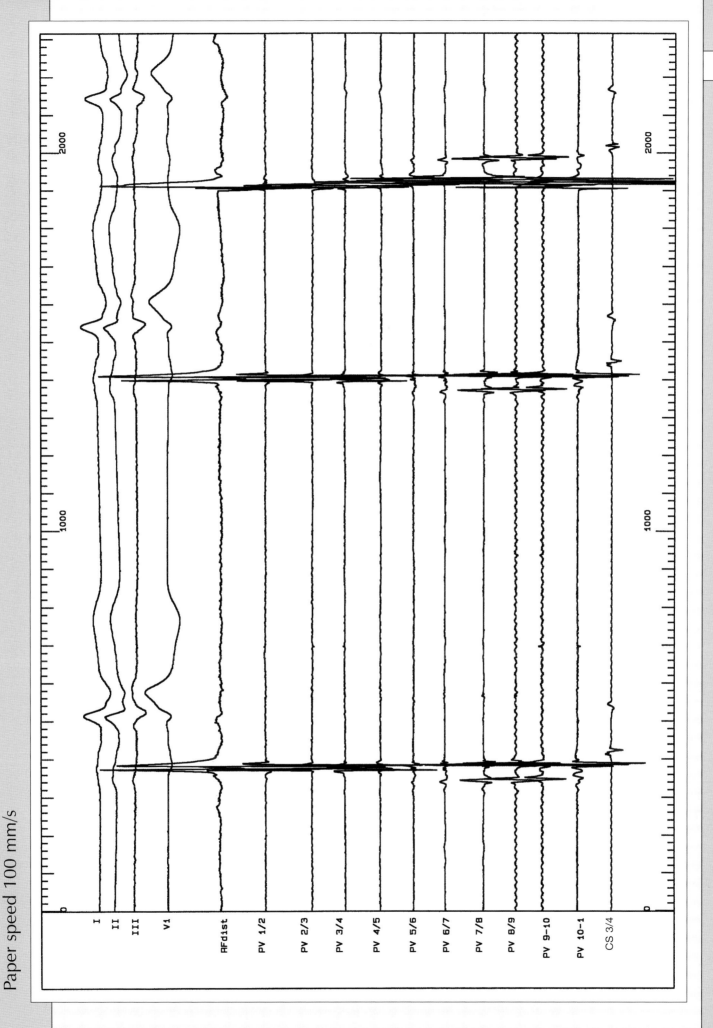

- There is reversal of the atrium (A) to PV (✱) activation sequence with the third beat, representing an ectopic beat of PV origin with local activation preceding the surface P wave (arrow and dotted line). The P-wave morphology of the ectopic beat is similar to that seen in sinus rhythm, which is consistent with ectopy from the RSPV or SVC. Because there is no clear activation sequence of the PVP, polarity reversal can be used as a guide to commence ablation by reducing the amplification of the PV signals.

Paper speed 100 mm/s

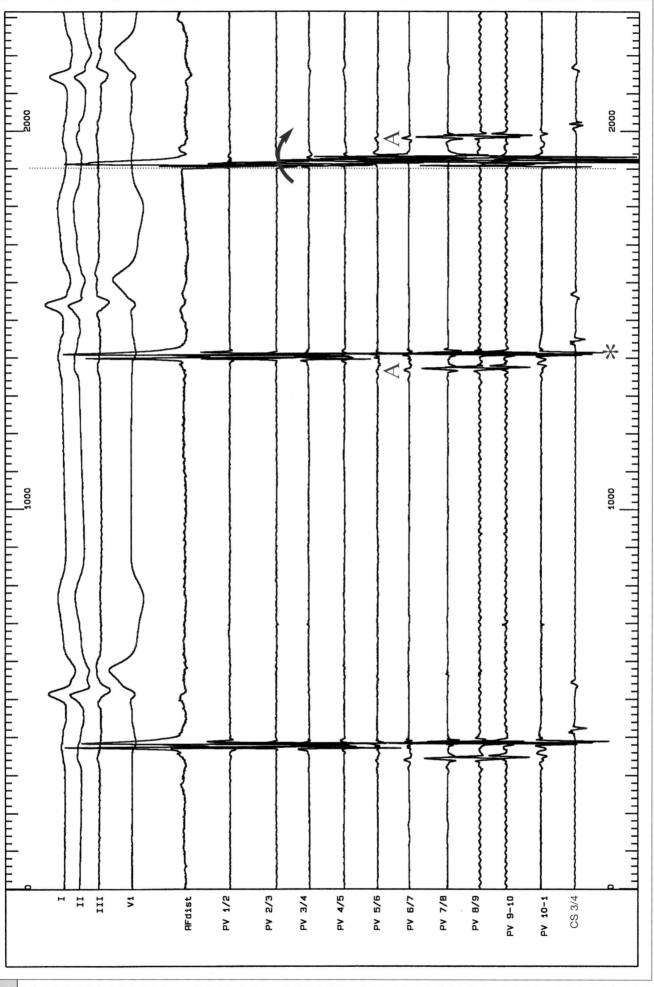

- This tracing is from an LSPV (the LASSO shaft is at the top of the vein).

  Where is the breakthrough?

Paper speed 100 mm/s

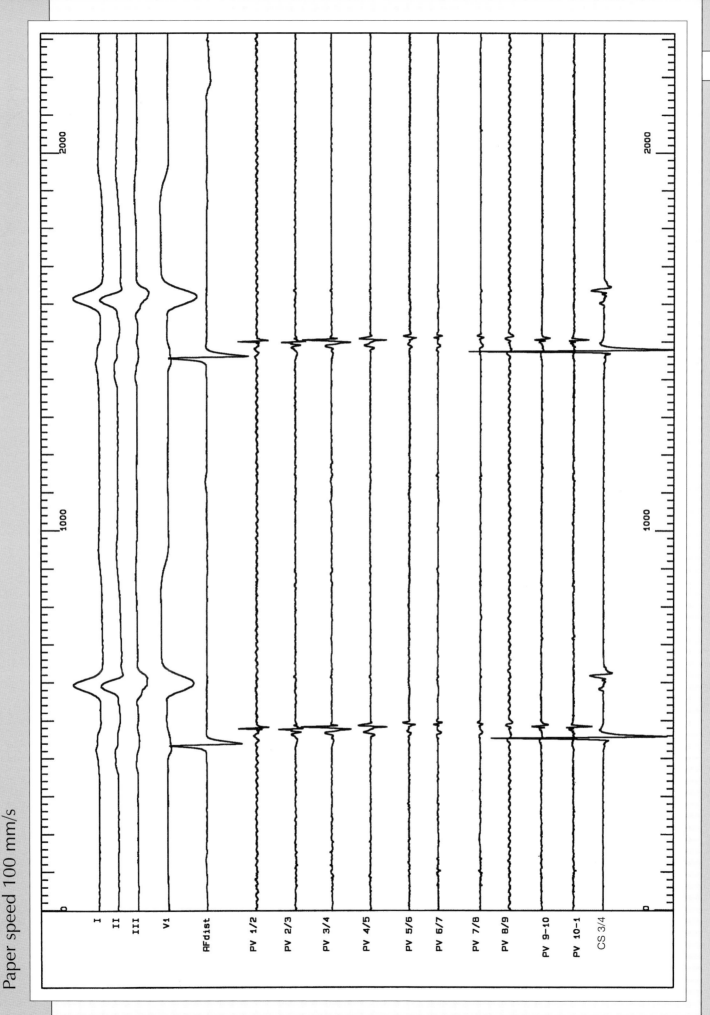

CASE 16 PART 2

- There is spontaneous delayed conduction between the LA and PV, meaning that the PVP (∗) can be distinguished from the atrial far-field signal (A), even in sinus rhythm. The breakthrough is at LASSO pole 9.

  What other maneuvers may be useful in confirming the breakthrough?

Paper speed 100 mm/s

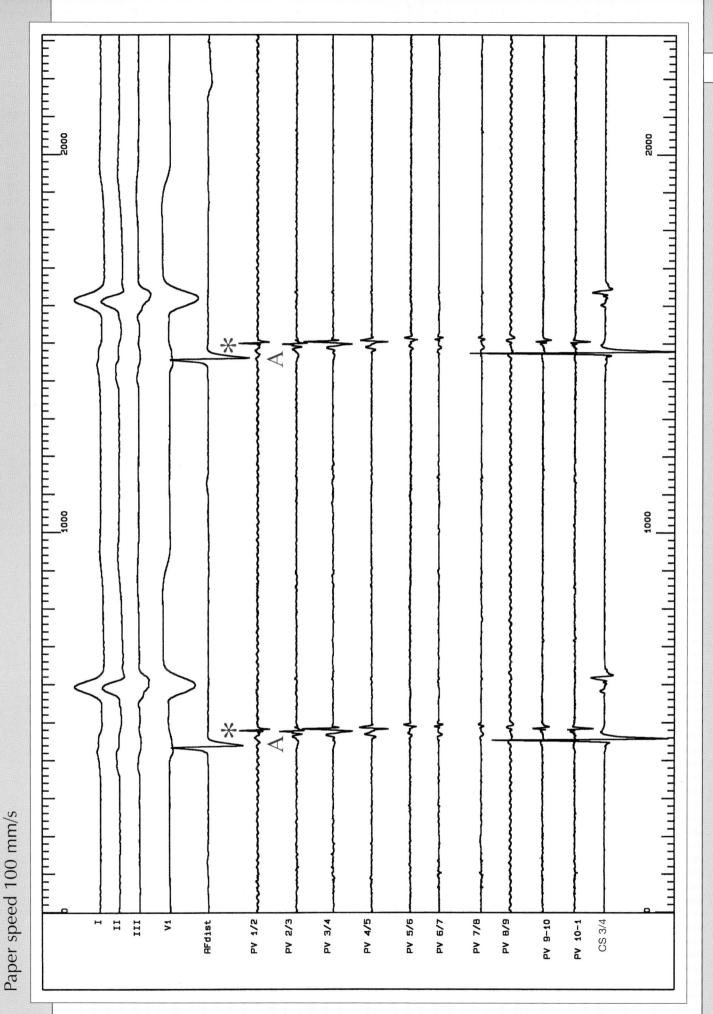

CASE 16 PART 3

- Pacing the CS (as in this tracing) or the LAA would separate the PVP and atrial far-field signals and confirm the breakthrough at LASSO pole 9 (* and dotted line). Sometimes, a different breakthrough is identified during sinus rhythm compared with CS pacing.

Paper speed 100 mm/s

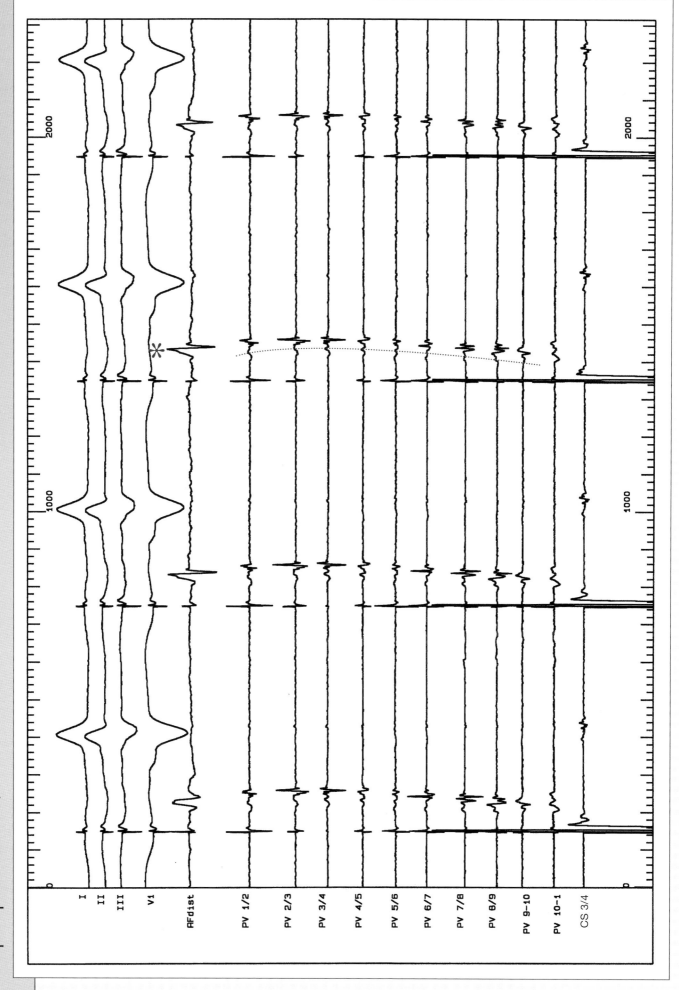

- This is the same patient during AFIB.

Where is the breakthrough?

Paper speed 100 mm/s

I
II
III
V1
AFdist
PV 1/2
PV 2/3
PV 3/4
PV 4/5
PV 5/6
PV 6/7
PV 7/8
PV 8/9
PV 9-10
PV 10-1
CS 3/4

2000

1000

0

CASE 16 PART 5

- The patient is now in AFIB with organized activity (✳) in the PV, confirming again that the main breakthrough is at the top of the vein (pole 9–10). Note that the LA far-field signal (A), which has a 1:1 association with the venous potentials, can be identified on the LASSO recording.

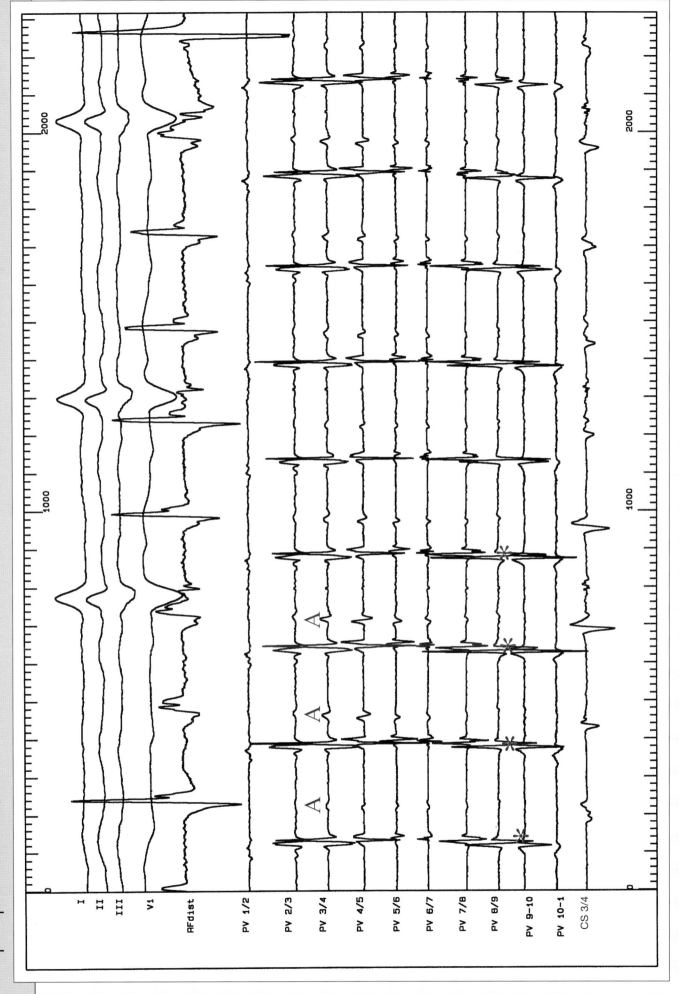

Paper speed 100 mm/s

CASE 16 PART 6

- This tracing is recorded following ablation of the LSPV.

  Is the vein disconnected?

Paper speed 100 mm/s

I

II

III

V1

AFdist

PV 1/2

PV 2/3

PV 3/4

PV 4/5

PV 5/6

PV 6/7

PV 7/8

PV 8/9

PV 9-10

PV 10-1

CS 3/4

2000

1000

CASE 16 PART 7

- During CS pacing, activity is recorded from the anterior part of the vein. This is the most common site for an LA far-field signal, as the LAA is anterior to the LSPV.

  The next trace shows LASSO recordings during LAA pacing, confirming that these signals represent LAA far-field signals.

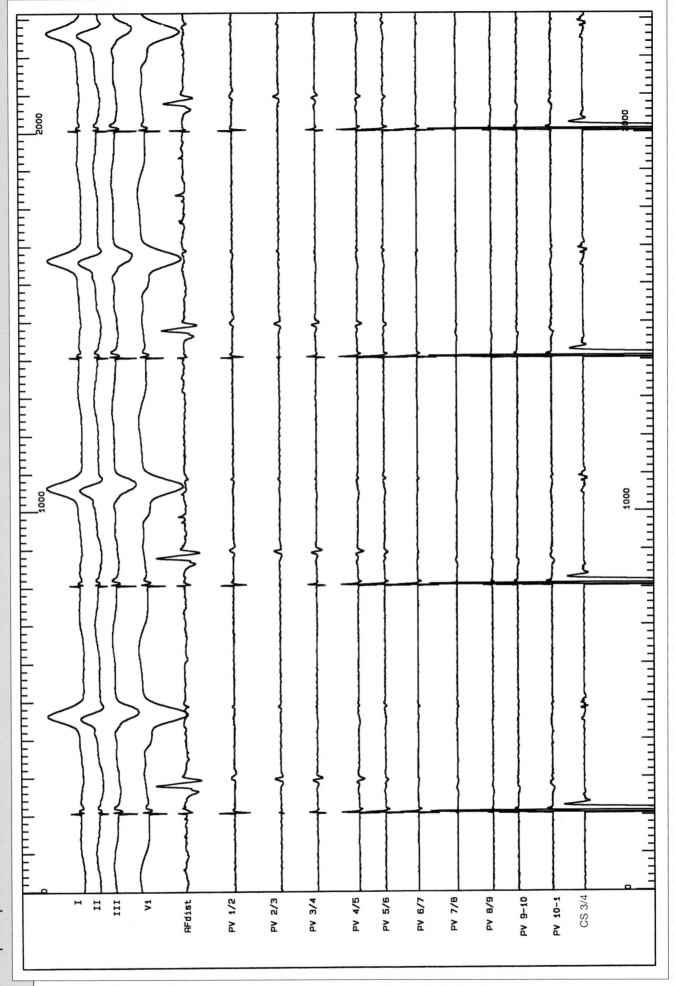

CASE 16 PART 8

- Pacing the LAA using the mapping catheter anticipates the LASSO signals (arrow), confirming that they are far-field signals from the LAA, and not PVPs. Therefore, the vein is disconnected.

Paper speed 100 mm/s

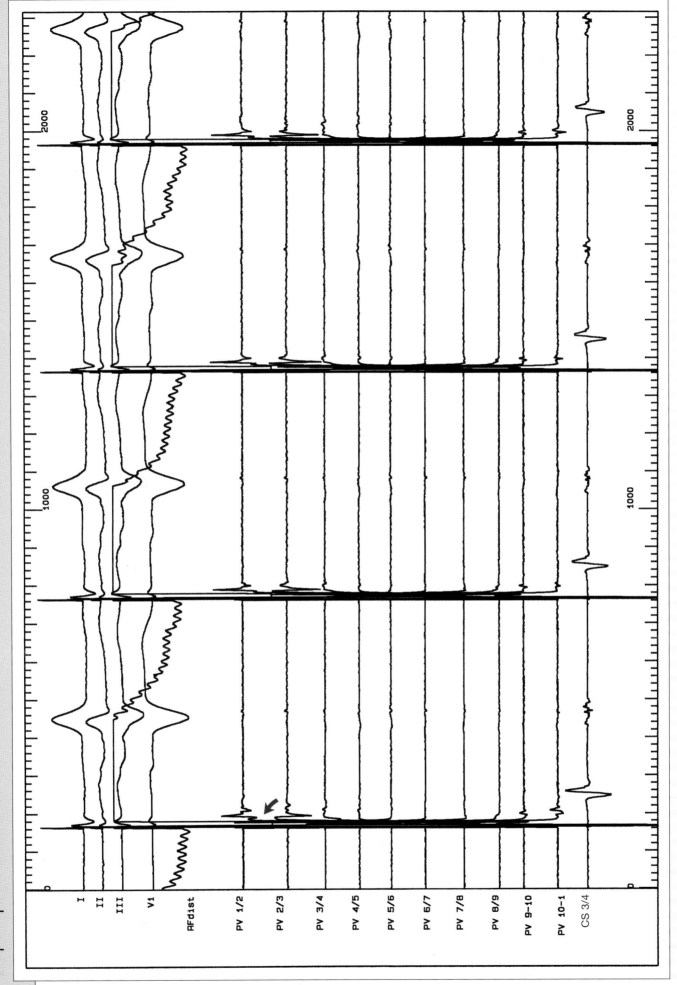

CASE 17 PART 1

- This tracing is from an LIPV (the LASSO shaft is at the top of the vein).

  What is the ablation target?

  What is your interpretation of the signals marked with the unfilled and solid arrows?

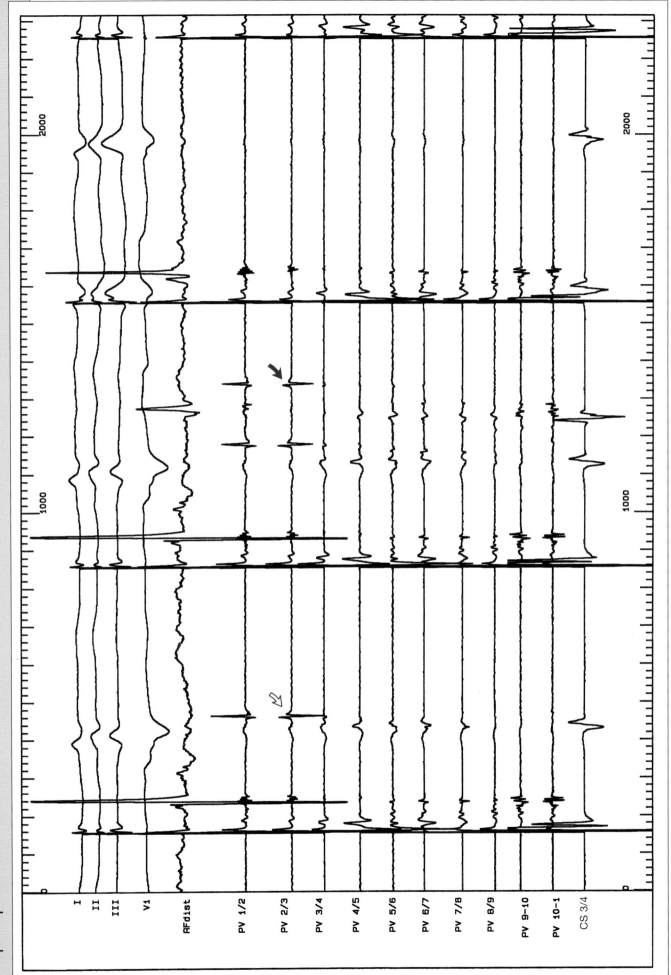

Paper speed 100 mm/s

CASE 17 PART 2

- The PVP is fractionated and of low amplitude due to previous RF ablation. The ablation target is LASSO bipole 10–1, as the earliest activity is here. The unfilled arrow indicates a concealed PV discharge from pole 1, while the solid arrow indicates a conducted PV discharge from the same focus. Following this, there is another concealed discharge (light red arrow). Note the polarity reversal of this signal. A indicates the LAA far-field signal.

Paper speed 100 mm/s

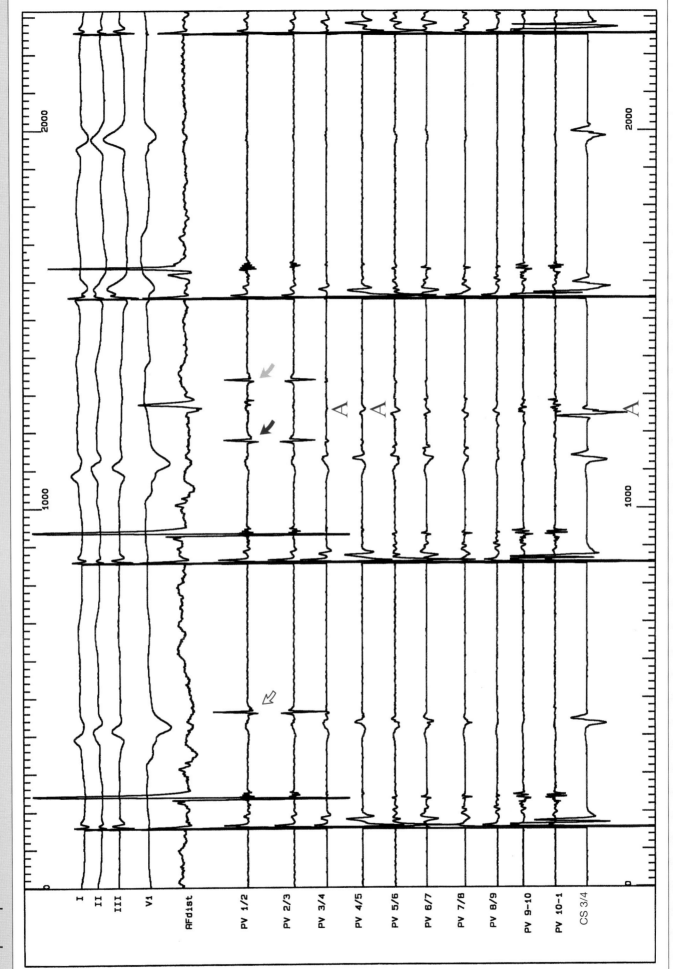

CASE 18 PART 1

- This LASSO tracing is from the LSPV (the LASSO shaft is at the posterior part of the vein) during a re-do case.

Where would you ablate?

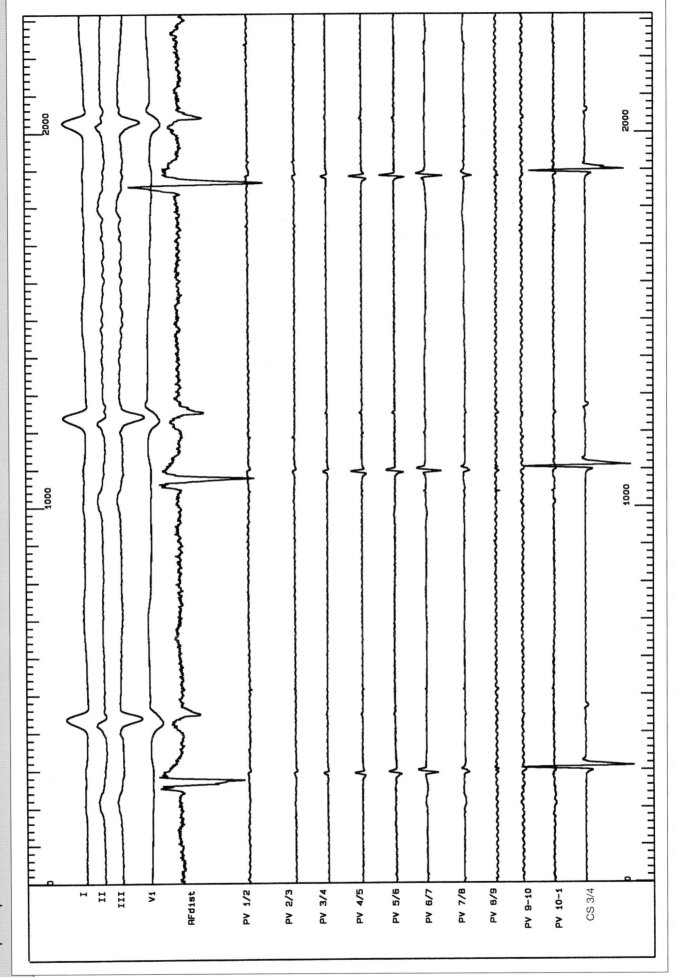

Paper speed 100 mm/s

147

CASE 18 PART 2

- The first step is to make sure that the signals represent PVPs (✱), rather than far-field signals. During CS pacing, note that the mapping signal lines up with the LASSO signal (dotted line) when the mapping catheter is placed in the LAA. When the shaft is posterior, LASSO poles 3–6 represent the anterior wall, which should make you even more suspicious that this is a far-field signal.

Paper speed 100 mm/s

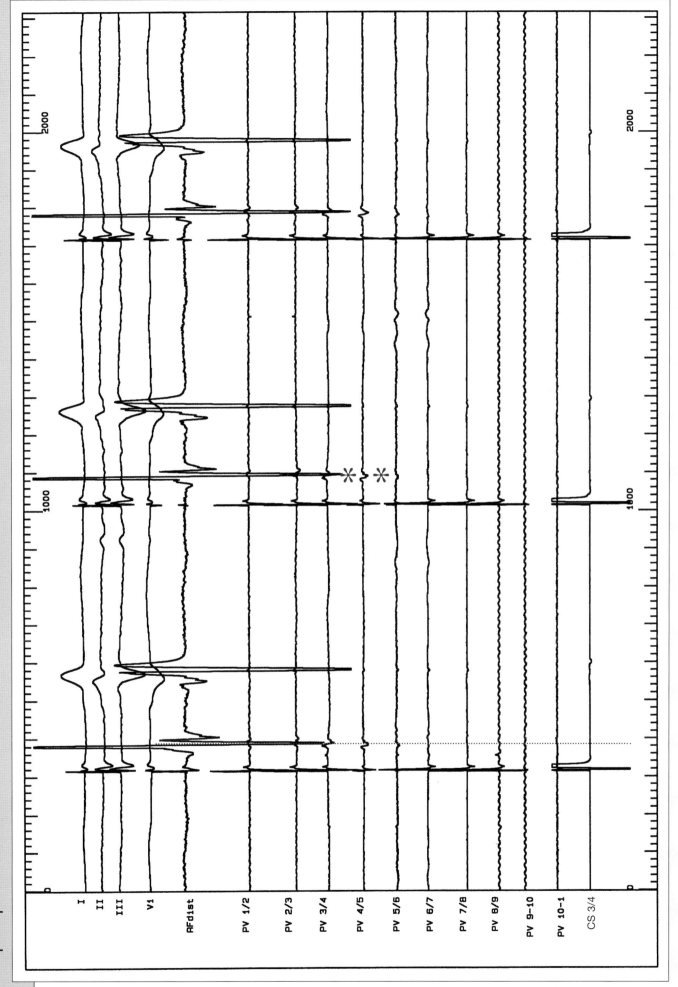

- Pacing the mapping catheter in the LAA confirms that the signals (✳) are far-field, as they are advanced by pacing, and ablation is not required in this vein.

Paper speed 100 mm/s

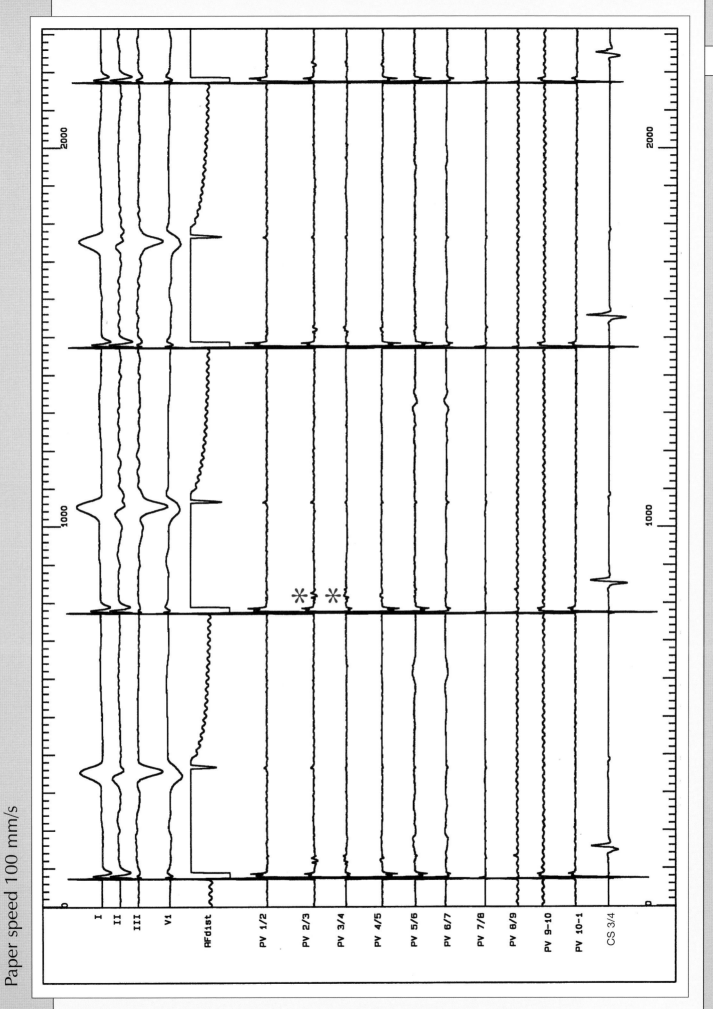

- This tracing is from an LSPV.

  What phenomenon is demonstrated?

  (Note: pacing from distal CS.)

Paper speed 100 mm/s

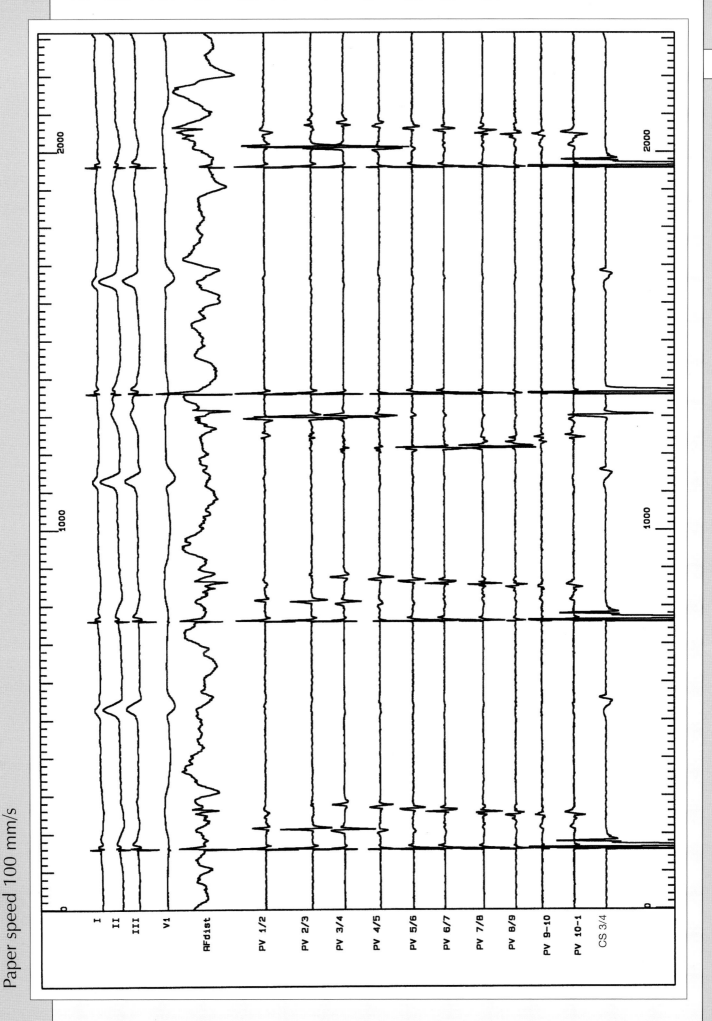

I
II
III
V1
AFdist
PV 1/2
PV 2/3
PV 3/4
PV 4/5
PV 5/6
PV 6/7
PV 7/8
PV 8/9
PV 9-10
PV 10-1
CS 3/4

2000
1000

2000
1000

CASE 19 PART 2

- There is reversal of the activation sequence during the third beat (dotted box), such that PV activity (∗) precedes LA (A). It is likely that the signals recorded on LASSO poles 1–3 (solid box) are LAA far-field signals as they are recorded at the anterior part of the vein; however, it would be valuable to confirm this by LAA pacing.

Paper speed 100 mm/s

I
II
III
V1
RFdist
PV 1/2
PV 2/3
PV 3/4
PV 4/5
PV 5/6
PV 6/7
PV 7/8
PV 8/9
PV 9–10
PV 10–1
CS 3/4

1000

2000

CASE 20 PART 1

- This is a 12-lead ECG from a patient returning 1 month after 4-PV isolation for the treatment of AFIB ablation. The patient has experienced worsening palpitations – which are now even worse than they were before the procedure – as well as decreased effort tolerance, dizziness, and presyncope.

What is the diagnosis?

Paper speed 25 mm/s

CASE 20 PART 2

- This is an atypical flutter (✱), which, due to the history of previous ablation and atypical ECG morphology, is probably an LA flutter. LA flutter complicates PV isolation in 3%–5% of cases, presumably because ostial ablation creates large anatomical conduction barriers. Common circuits are perimitral and around the right or left ostia. In this case, mapping reveals perimitral re-entry. The ablation target is the isthmus of tissue between the LIPV and lateral mitral annulus.

Paper speed 25 mm/s

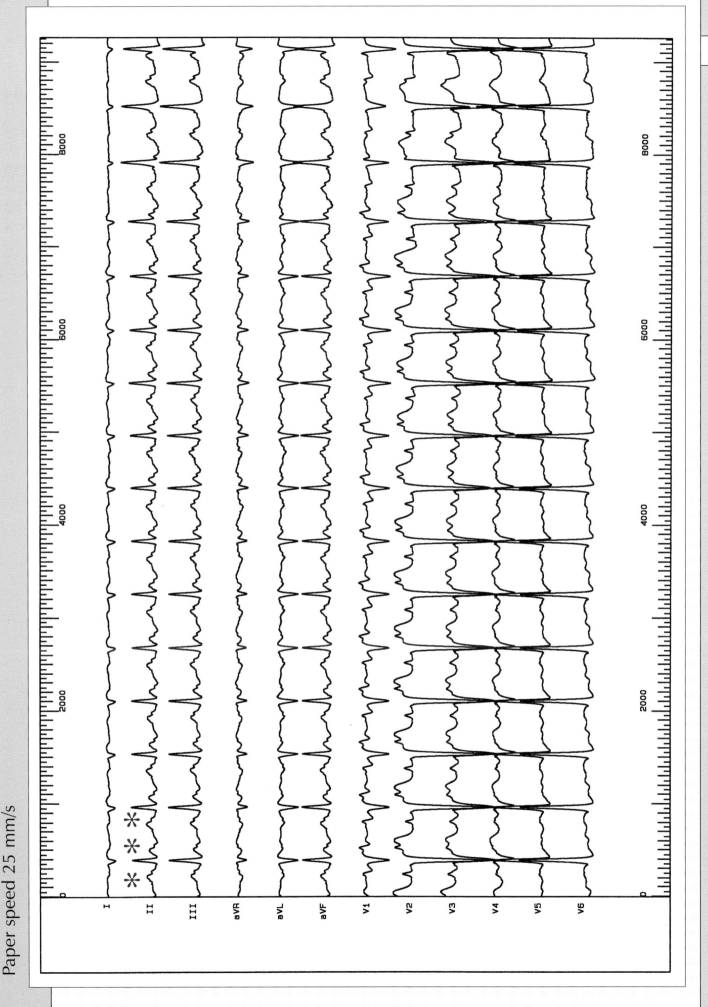

CASE 20 PART 3

- This is the mapping signal at the ablation site between the LIPV and the lateral mitral annulus. Proximal to distal activation in the CS suggests counterclockwise perimitral flutter. The mapping catheter records a fractionated mid-diastolic potential (between two flutter waves; dotted line), indicating an area of slow conduction (✳). Entrainment mapping (not shown) is also useful in cases such as this. Ablation at this site was successful (line between LIPV and MV).

Paper speed 100 mm/s

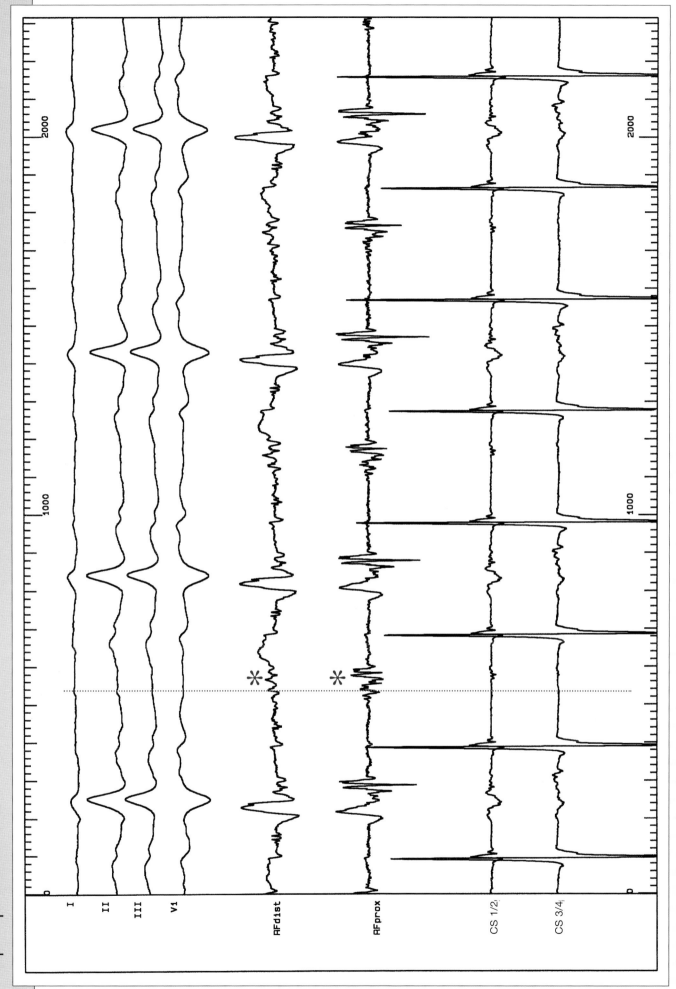

CASE 21 PART 1

- After PV isolation, the right veins were checked. In this case, the LASSO is in the RSPV while the mapping catheter is within the RIPV.

Are the signals recorded on the LASSO PVP or far-field?

Paper speed 100 mm/s

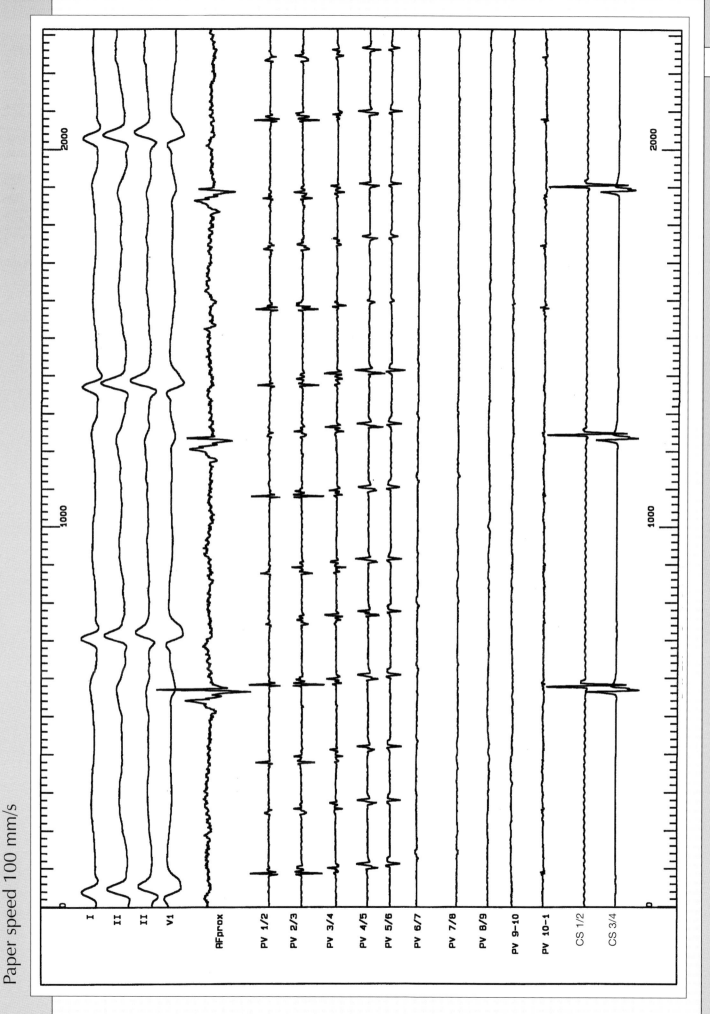

CASE 21 PART 2

- The tracing shows dissociated PV activity "firing" (★), whereas the LA is in sinus rhythm (note CS atrial signals and surface ECG). Far-field signals are usually of very low amplitude in the right veins. The mapping catheter records conduction recovery within the RIPV (✳). The LASSO should be moved to the RIPV to better define the ablation target.

Paper speed 100 mm/s

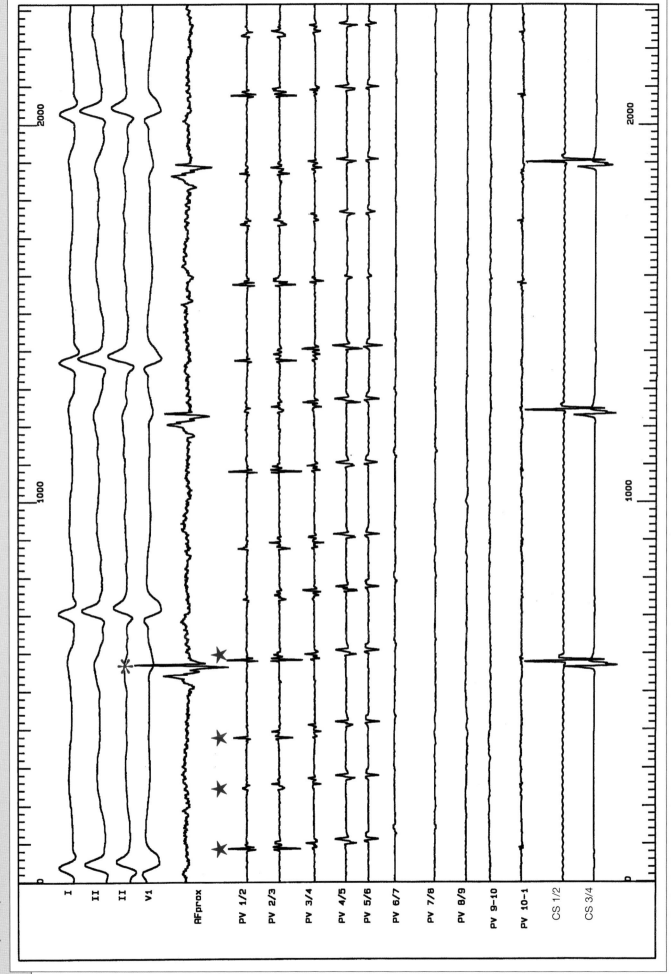

CASE 22 PART 1

- This tracing is from an LSPV during AFIB (the catheter is in the LSPV).

Is the rhythm organized or disorganized?

Paper speed 100 mm/s

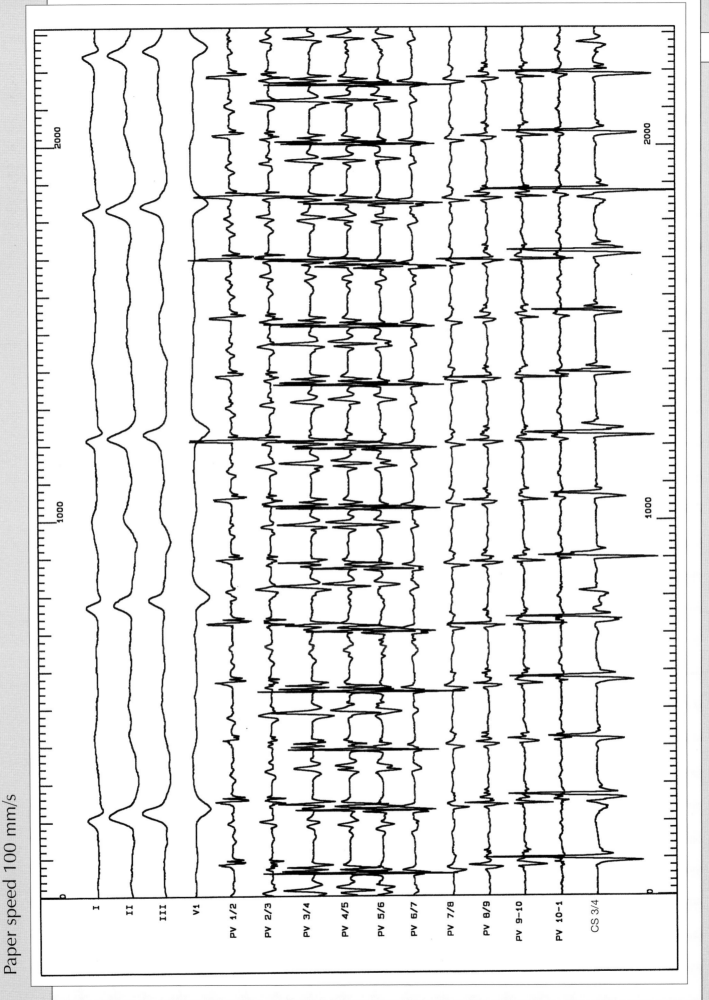

CASE 22 PART 2

- This is organized activity, with atrial far-field signals (A) distinct from the PVP (✻). The atrial far-field signal is most obvious in the anterior part of this vein. The sequence of PV activation is repetitive, with polarity reversal and the earliest activity at the bottom of the vein (dotted line).

Paper speed 100 mm/s

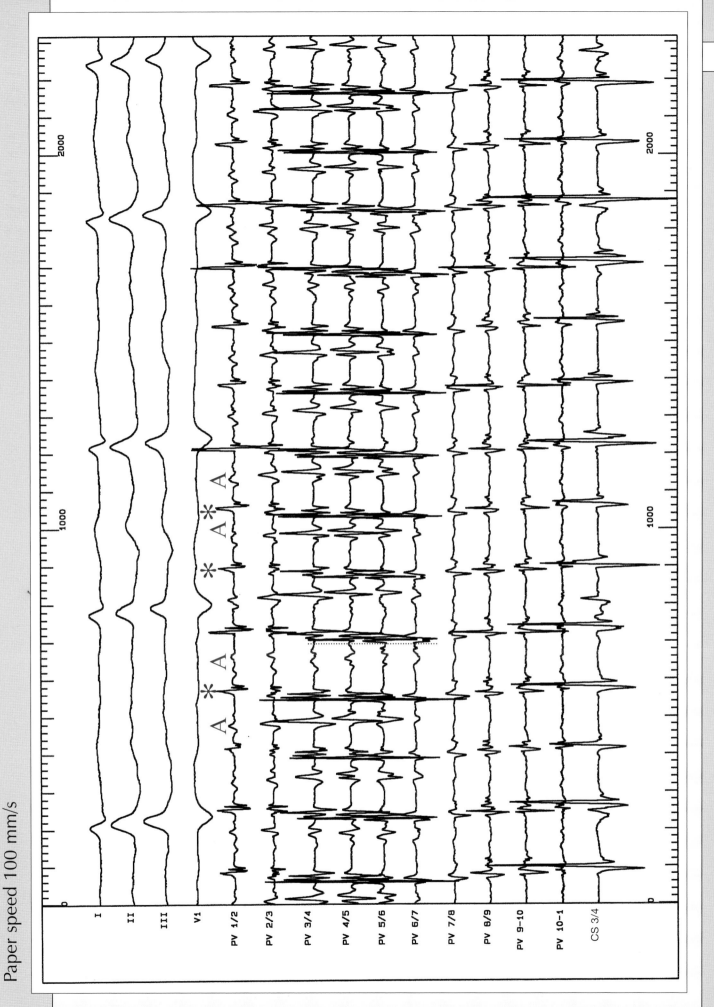

CASE 22 PART 3

- This is the same vein a few minutes later.

  What has changed?

Paper speed 100 mm/s

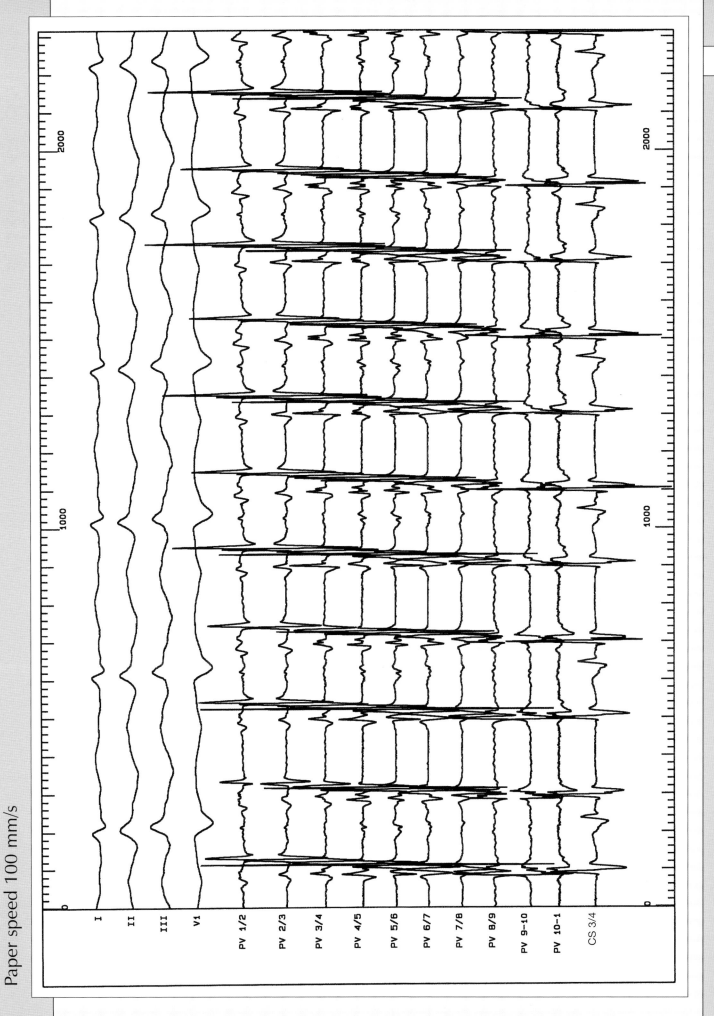

I

II

III

V1

PV 1/2

PV 2/3

PV 3/4

PV 4/5

PV 5/6

PV 6/7

PV 7/8

PV 8/9

PV 9-10

PV 10-1

CS 3/4

2000

1000

CASE 22 PART 4

- The patient is now in common flutter (surface ECG). The activation sequence in the PV (✱) is the same, and an LA far-field signal (A) can be seen preceding each PVP (1:1 activation into the LSPV).

Paper speed 100 mm/s

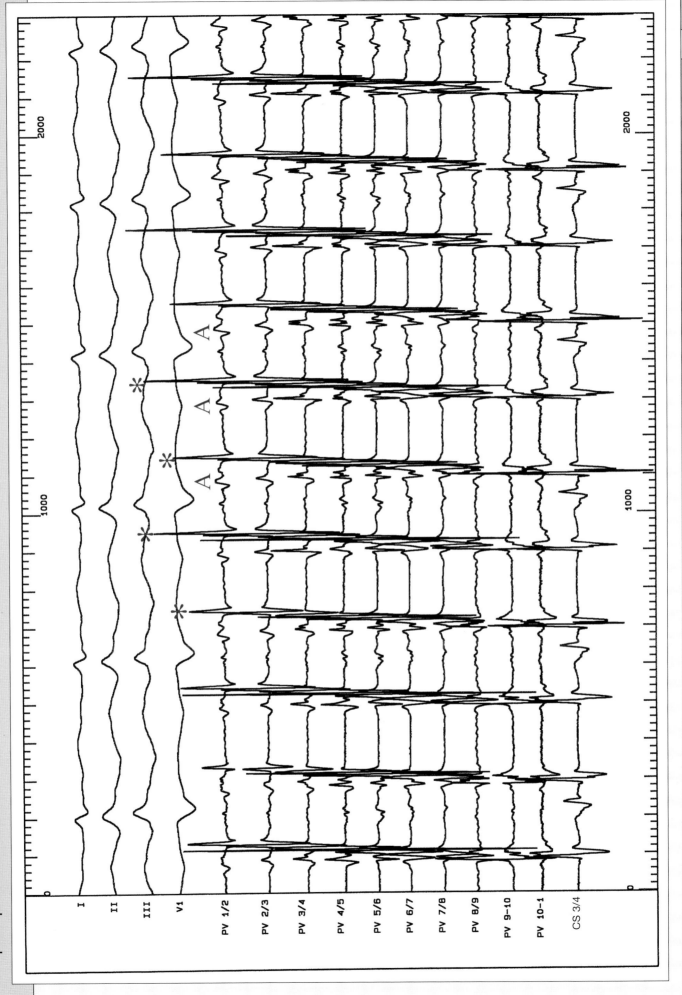

CASE 23 PART 1

- During a recurrence case, the following tracing is recorded on the mapping catheter (RF dist) from the bottom of the LIPV.

  Is ablation required at this site?

Paper speed 100 mm/s

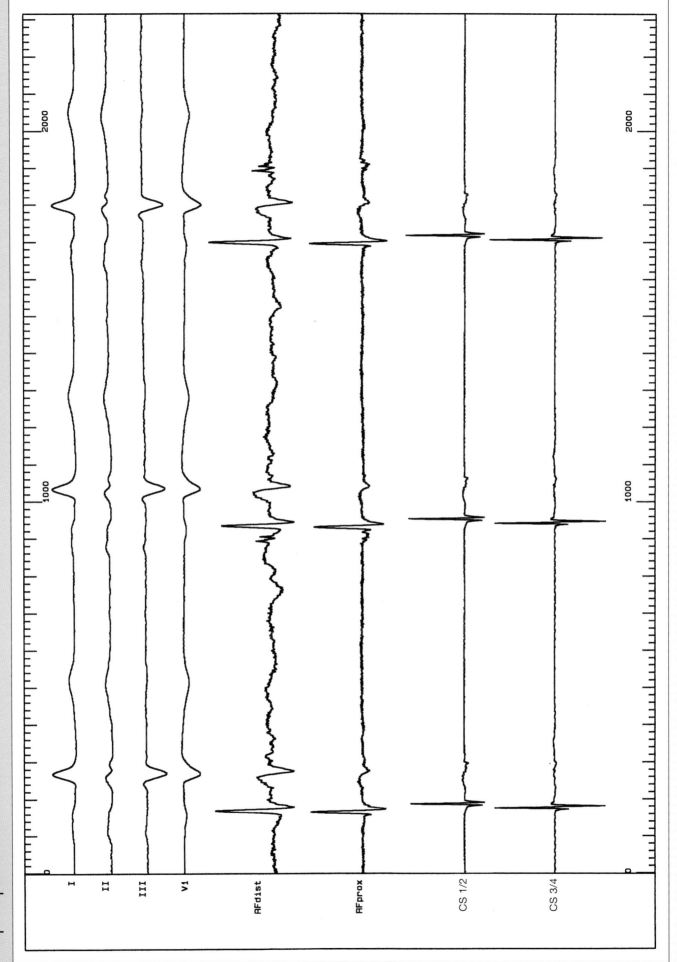

175

- The tracing demonstrates a dissociated PVP (∗). Ablation is not required at this site.

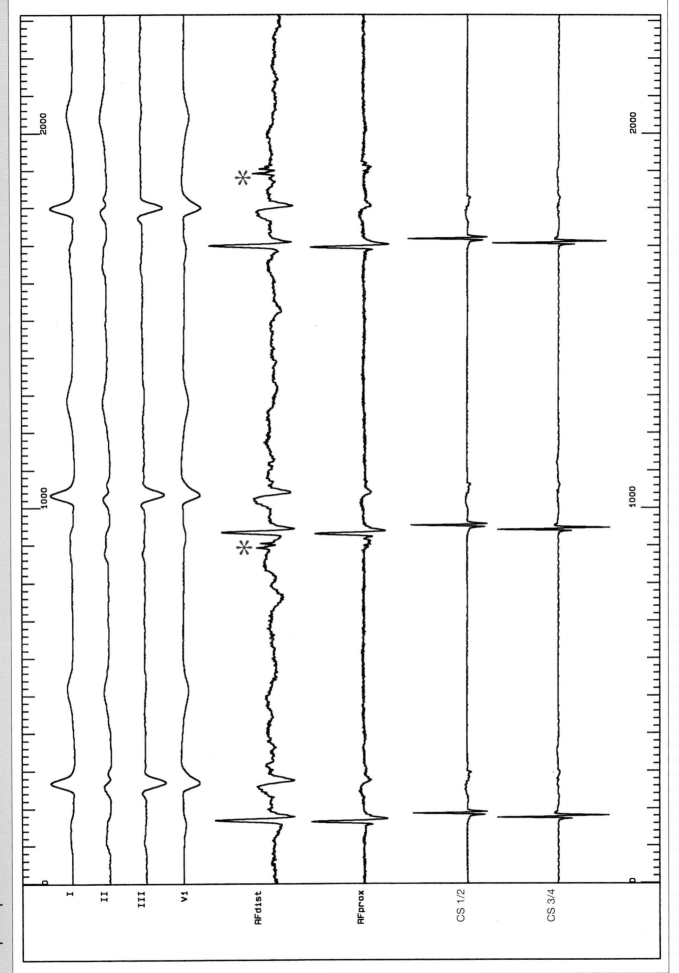

- Pacing the CS confirms dissociation of the PVP (*). "A" indicates the LAA far field. "S" indicates a stimulation artifact.

Paper speed 100 mm/s

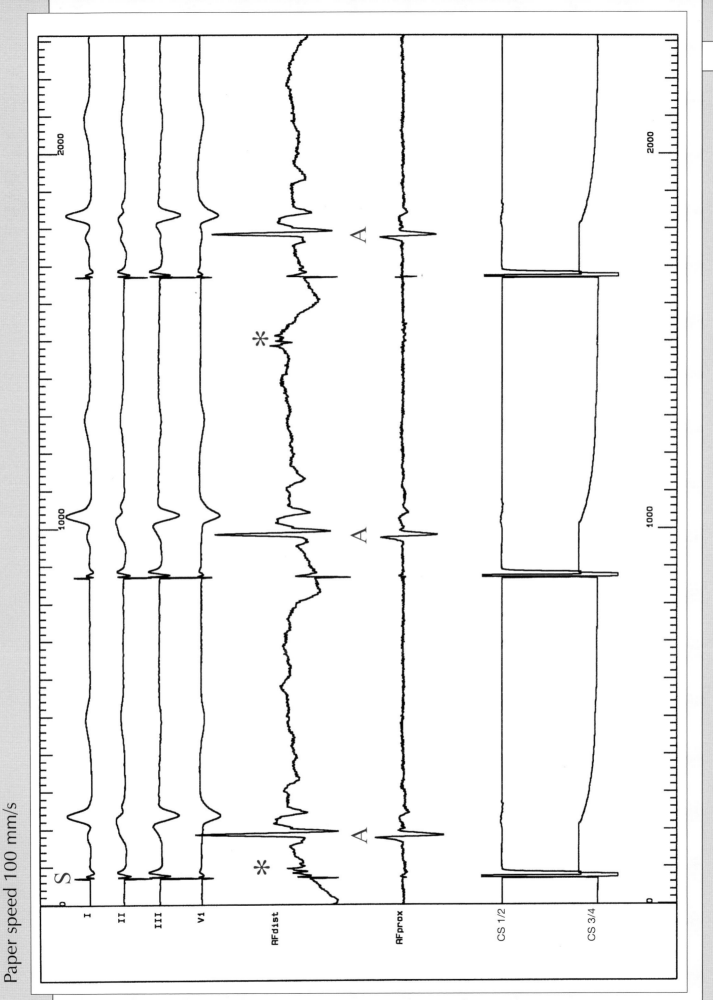

CASE 24 PART 1

- The next two tracings are from an RSPV (the LASSO shaft is at the top of the vein).

  Look at and provide an explanation for the activity of both.

Paper speed 100 mm/s

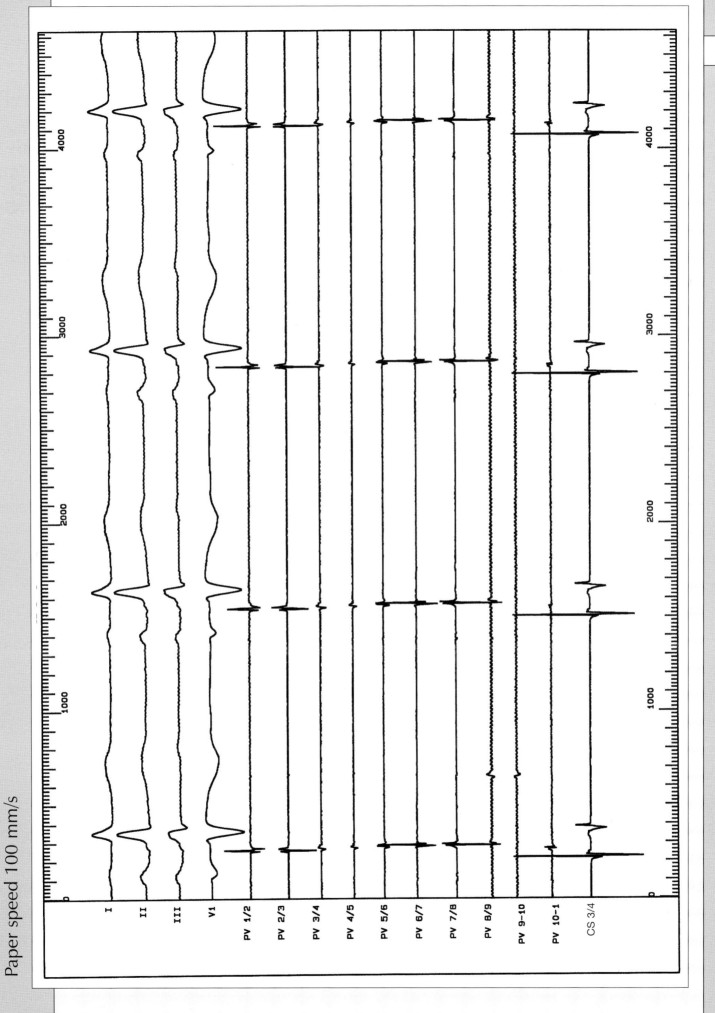

- The second tracing.

Paper speed 100 mm/s

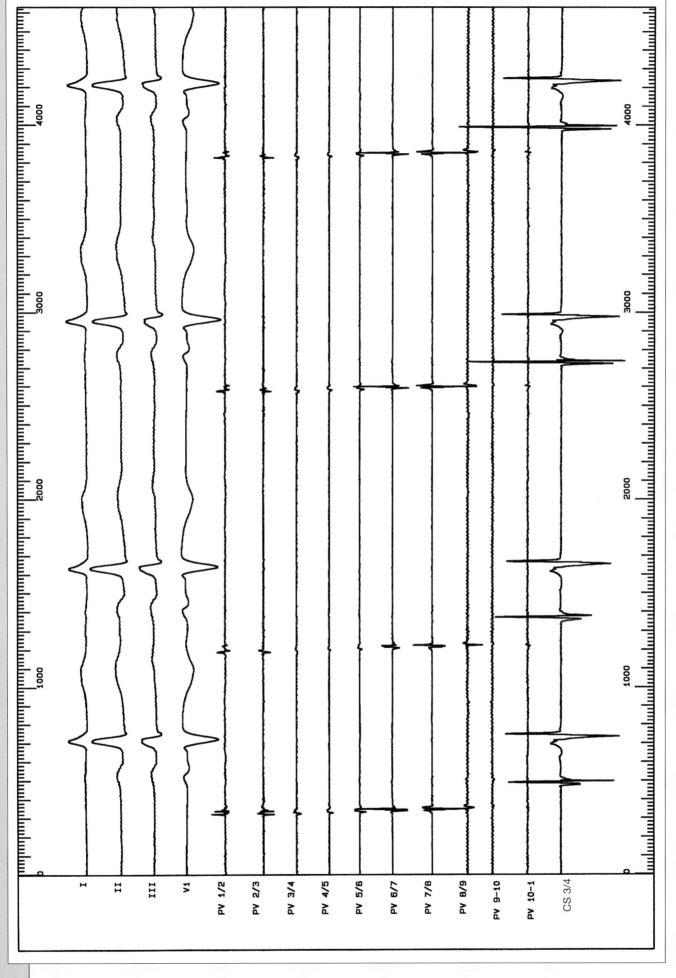

- The first tracing shows normal sinus rhythm, with passive activation of the PV demonstrated by CS activation (A) preceding PVP (✻). The earliest PVP is at LASSO pole 2.

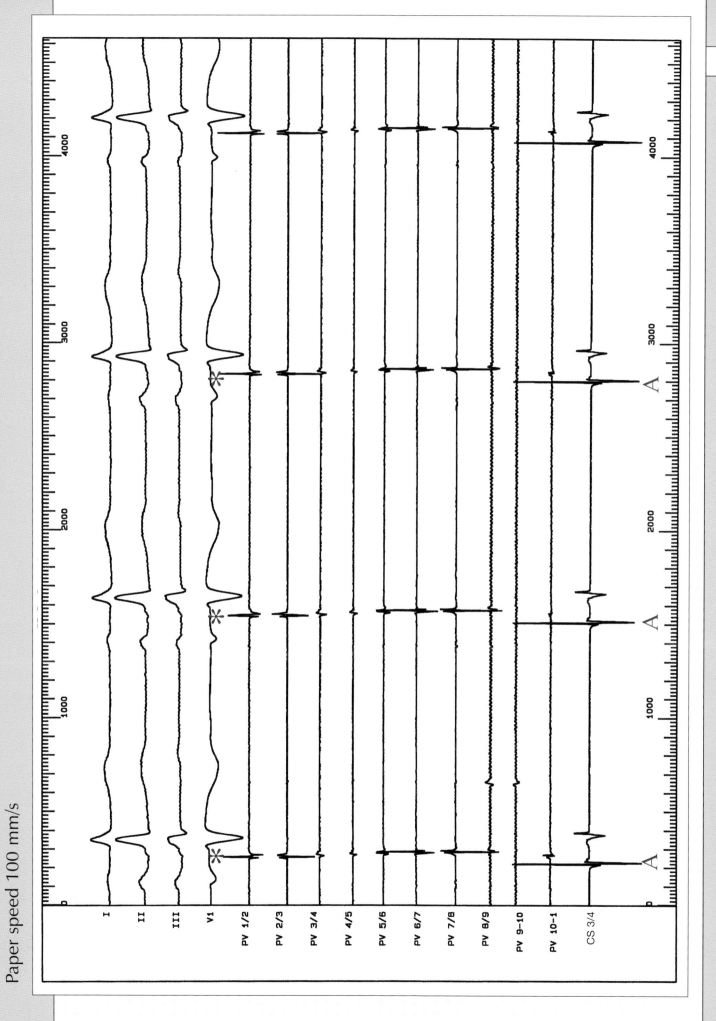

Paper speed 100 mm/s

185

CASE 24 PART 4

- The second tracing shows venous ectopy, which somewhat mimics sinus rhythm – except that the P wave in V1 is completely different, as is the activation sequence between PV (✶) and LA (A).

Paper speed 100 mm/s

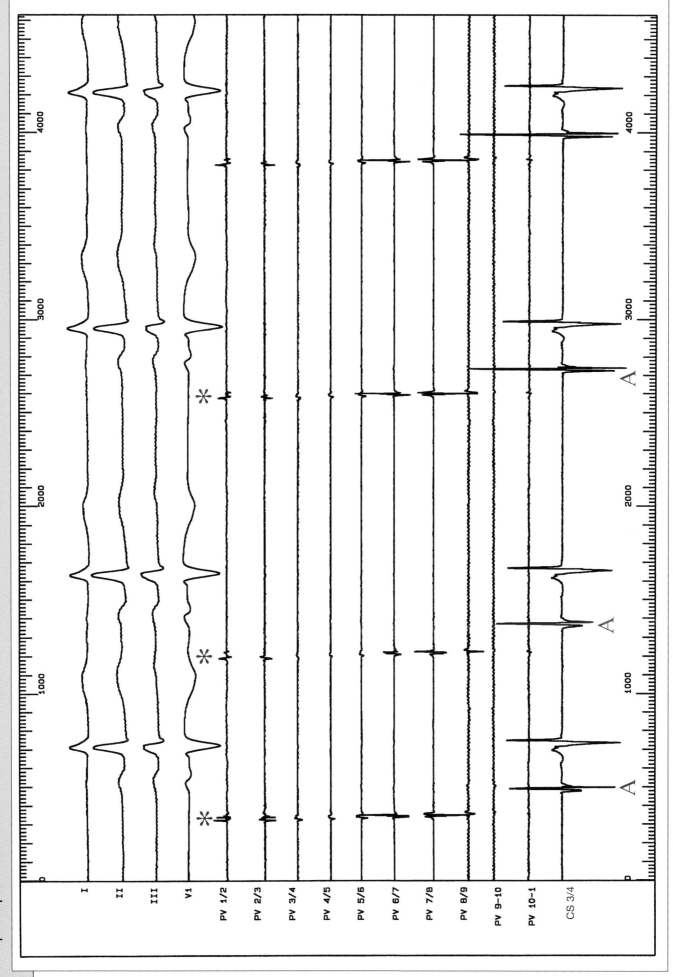

CASE 25 PART 1

- This shows a 12-lead ECG from a patient referred for AFIB ablation.

  Referring to the algorithm on page 45, where would you suspect the origin of this ectopy to be located?

Paper speed 25 mm/s

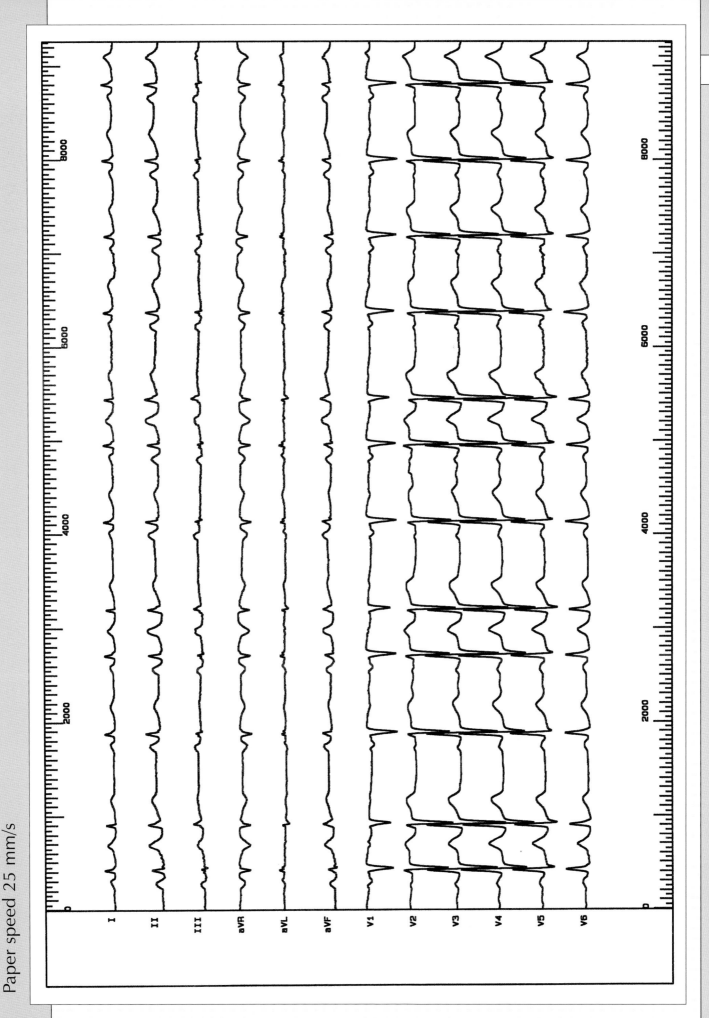

- The ectopic beat morphology is of amplitude ≥ 50 mV in lead I and >100 mV in lead II, consistent with an origin in or near the RSPV or the SVC. "p-on-T" ectopics can be seen (✳).

Paper speed 25 mm/s

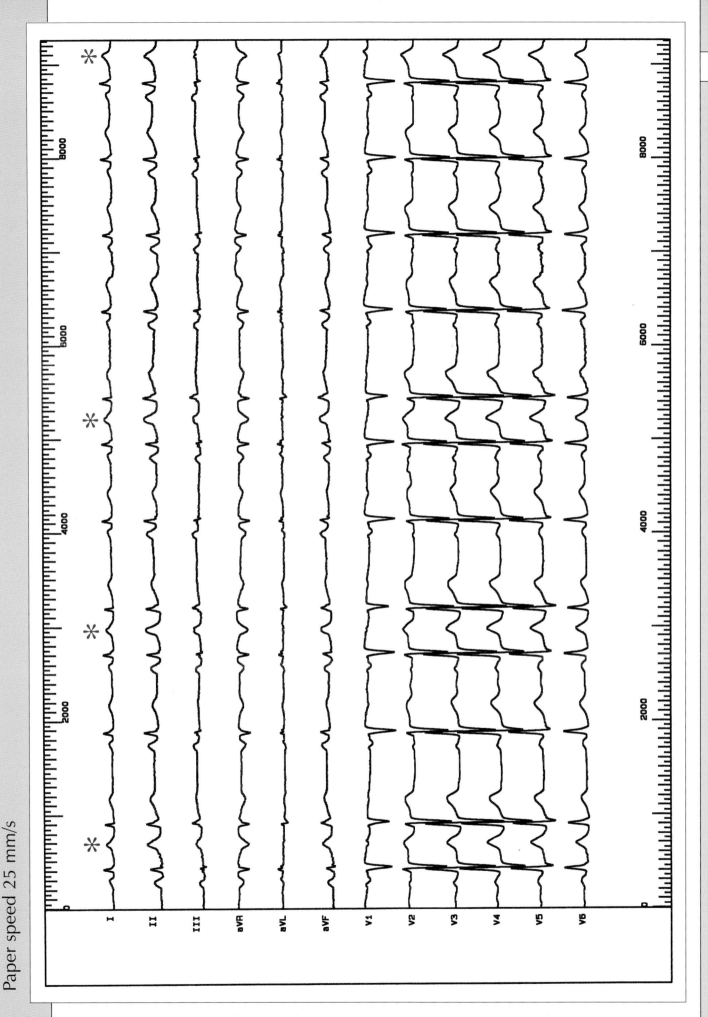

CASE 25 PART 3

- This is an RSPV LASSO recording in the same patient (the shaft is at the top of the vein).

  Where is the ablation target?

Paper speed 50 mm/s

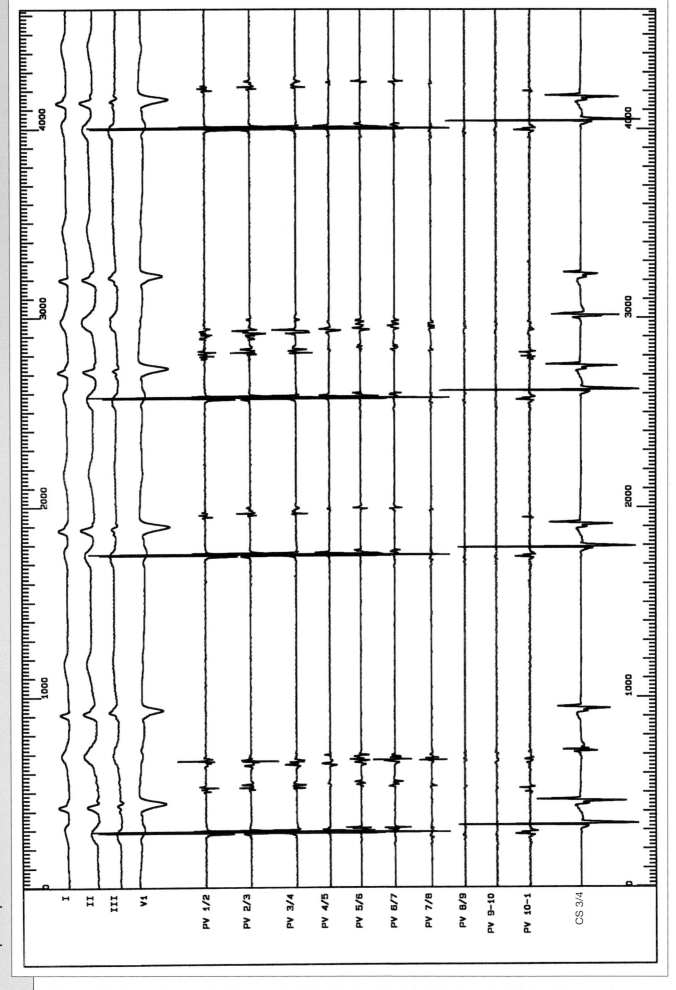

CASE 25 PART 4

- This tracing shows "p-on-T" atrial ectopic beats originating from the RSPV (arrow). The ablation target is LASSO pole 3, corresponding to the posterior wall of this vein; the earliest PVP is here, with polarity reversal.

Paper speed 50 mm/s

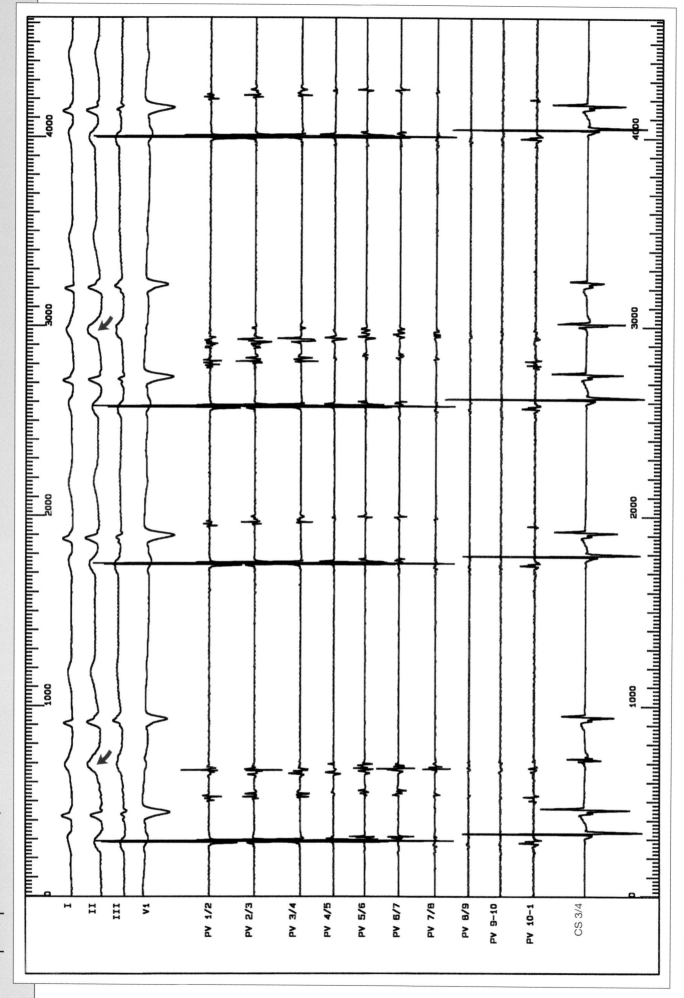

CASE 26 PART 1

- This tracing is from an LSPV during CS pacing (the LASSO shaft is at the top of the vein).

  What is your interpretation of the signals in the solid and dotted boxes?

Paper speed 100 mm/s

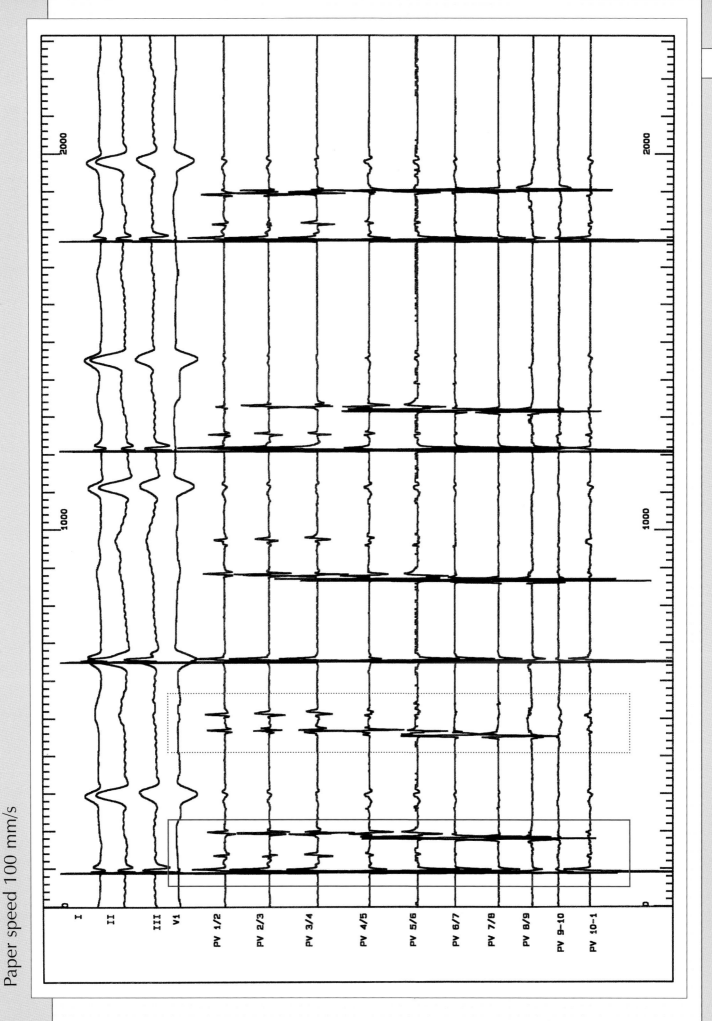

I
II
III
V1
PV 1/2
PV 2/3
PV 3/4
PV 4/5
PV 5/6
PV 6/7
PV 7/8
PV 8/9
PV 9-10
PV 10-1

2000

1000

- The signals in the solid box show atrium to PV activation, with LAA far-field signals recorded in the anterior part of the vein (A) (LASSO poles 1–4) and the earliest PVP (✳) in the posterior part of the vein.

  The dotted box shows PV ectopy with reversal of the activation sequence (A) and the same PV breakthrough (✳).

Paper speed 100 mm/s

CASE 26 PART 3

- This tracing was recorded during ablation in the same LSPV.

  What is your interpretation?

Paper speed 100 mm/s

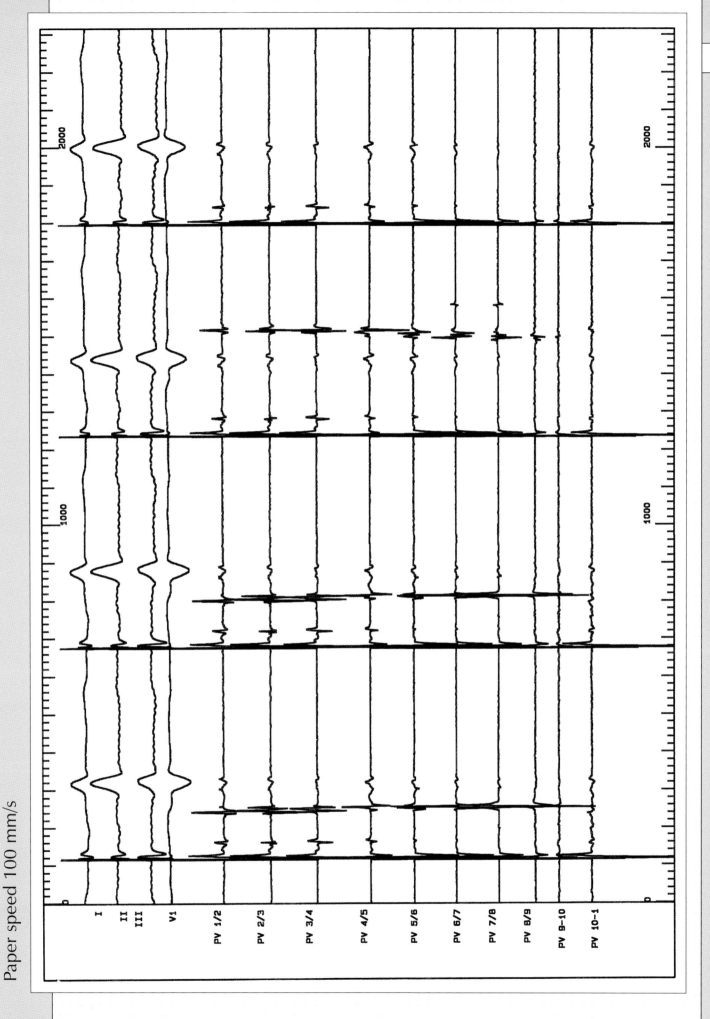

2000

1000

2000

1000

I

II

III

V1

PV 1/2

PV 2/3

PV 3/4

PV 4/5

PV 5/6

PV 6/7

PV 7/8

PV 8/9

PV 9-10

PV 10-1

CASE 26 PART 4

- The PV has been disconnected. Note the delay in the A to PVP interval caused by the ablation, as well as the change in the PV sequence compared with the earlier recording. Immediately prior to disconnection, there is a marked delay in the PVPs (arrow), presumably due to very slow conduction as a result of ablation.

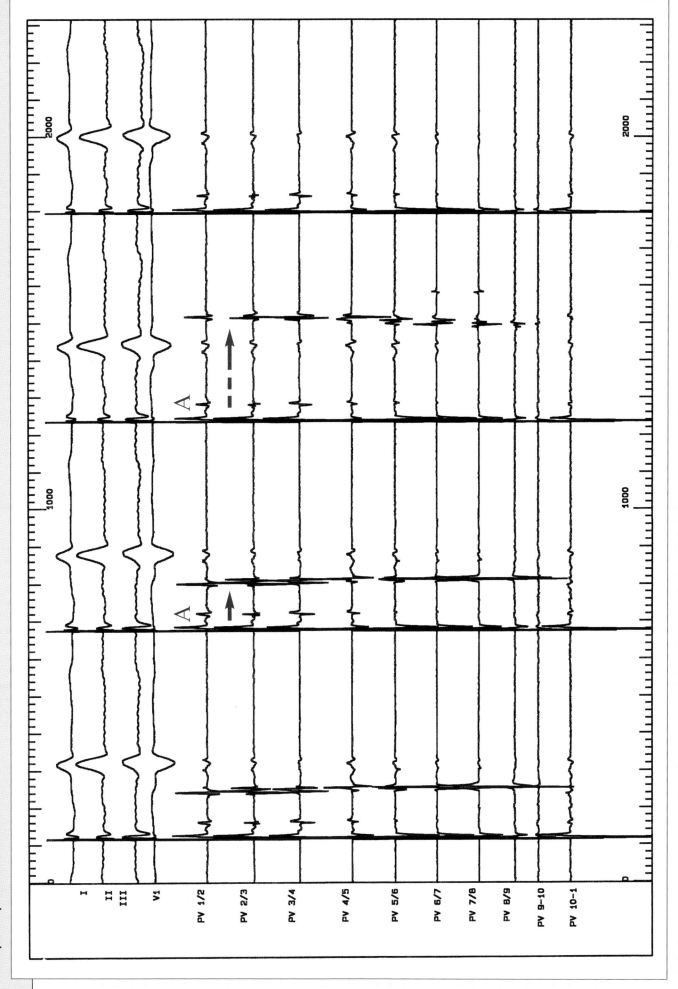

CASE 26 PART 5

- This is the same vein after ablation, showing dissociated PV activity (dotted boxes) and LAA far-field signals in the anterior part of the vein (solid box).

Paper speed 100 mm/s

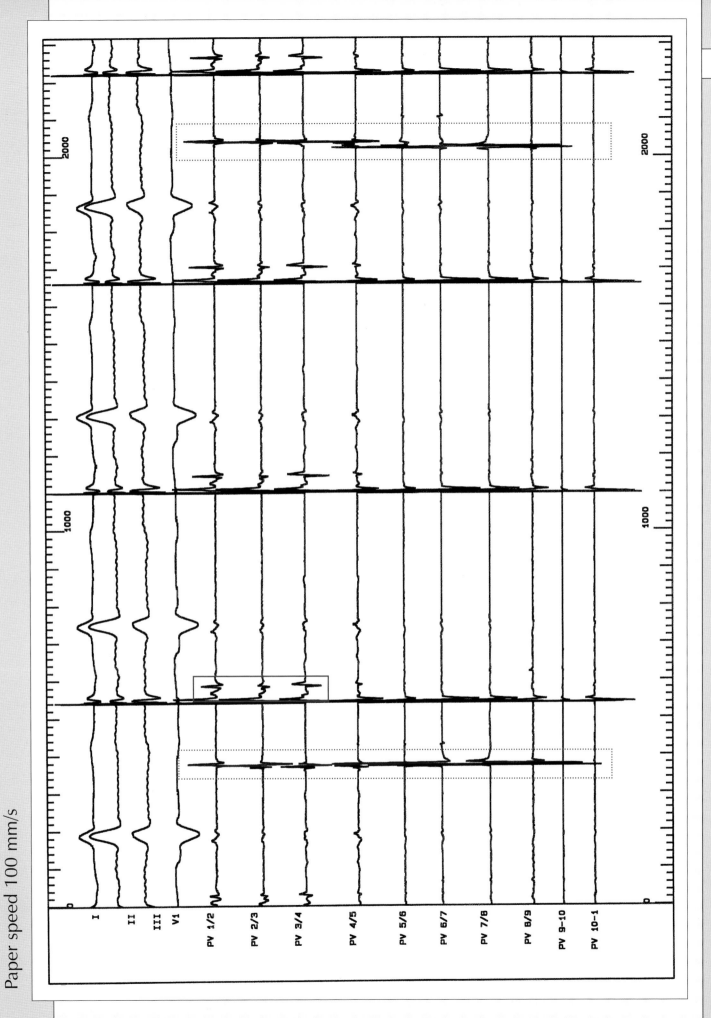

2000

1000

I
II
III
V1
PV 1/2
PV 2/3
PV 3/4
PV 4/5
PV 5/6
PV 6/7
PV 7/8
PV 8/9
PV 9-10
PV 10-1

CASE 27 PART 1

- This recording is from an LSPV during sinus rhythm prior to any ablation (the LASSO shaft is at the top posterior part of the vein).

Are any PVPs visible?

Paper speed 100 mm/s

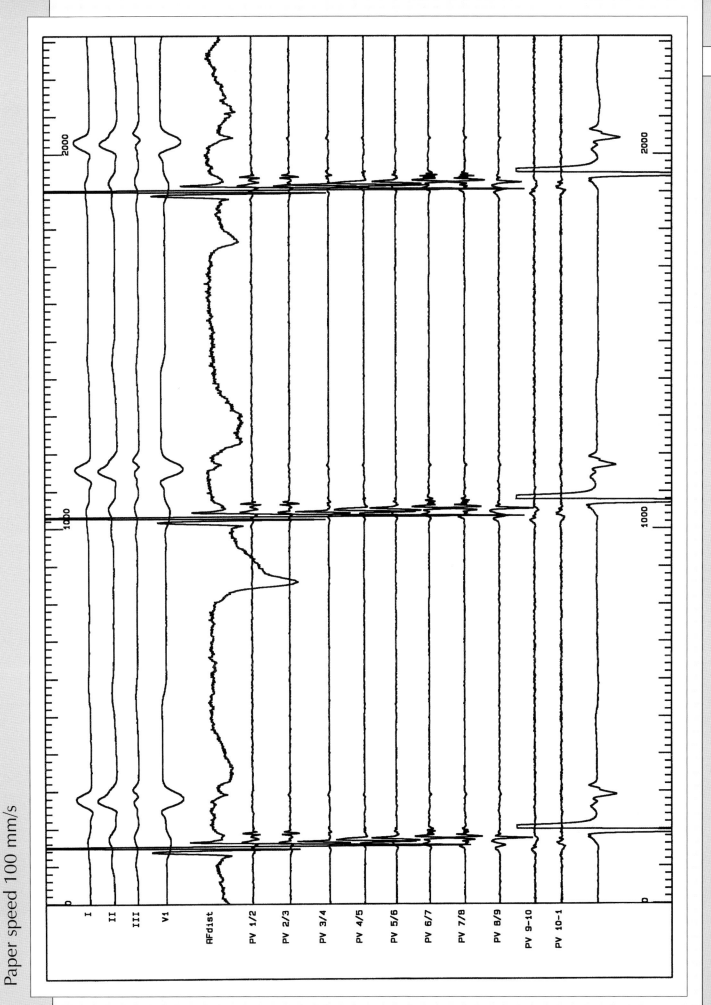

CASE 27 PART 2

- There probably are PVPs, as there are sharp potentials immediately following the LA signal (arrows). CS pacing would help to more clearly identify the PVP and the earliest breakthrough.

Paper speed 100 mm/s

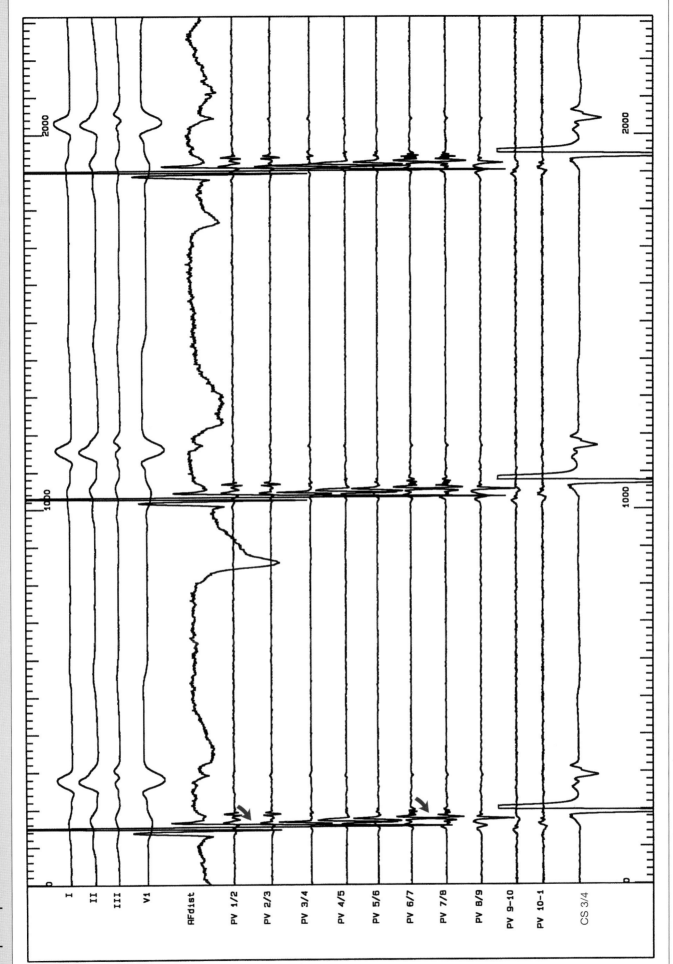

CASE 27 PART 3

- This is the same vein during distal CS pacing.

  In your opinion, where is the first target for ablation?

Paper speed 100 mm/s

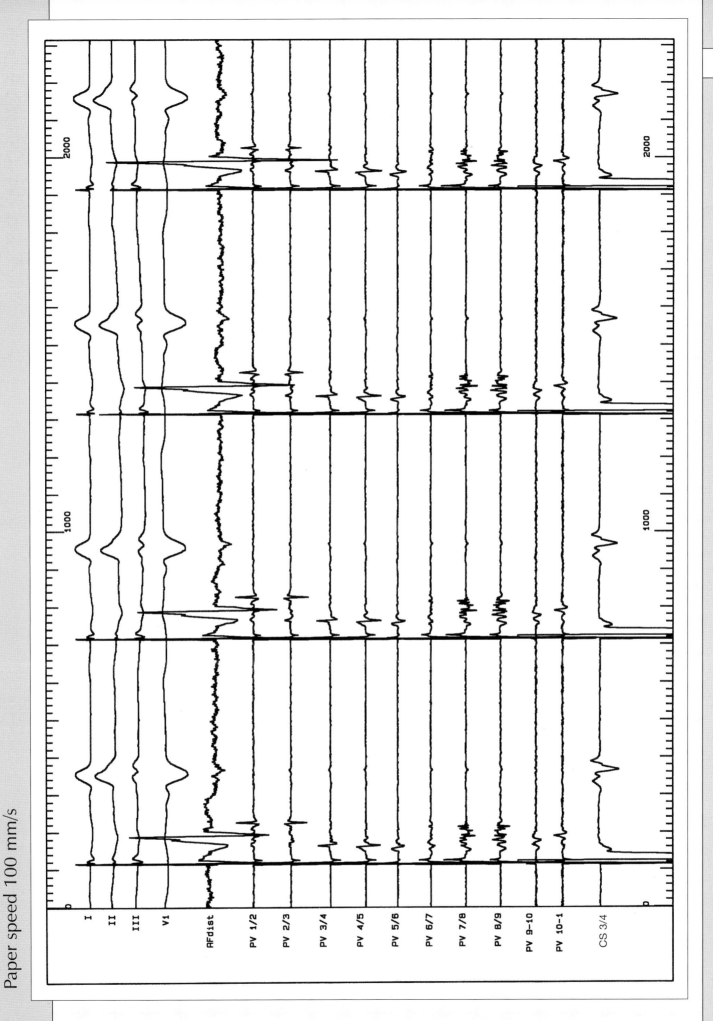

CASE 27 PART 4

- As expected, distal CS pacing clearly separates the LA and PVP signals, and the earliest PV breakthrough at LASSO pole 8 (✲) is now visible. The star (★) indicates the earliest activity.

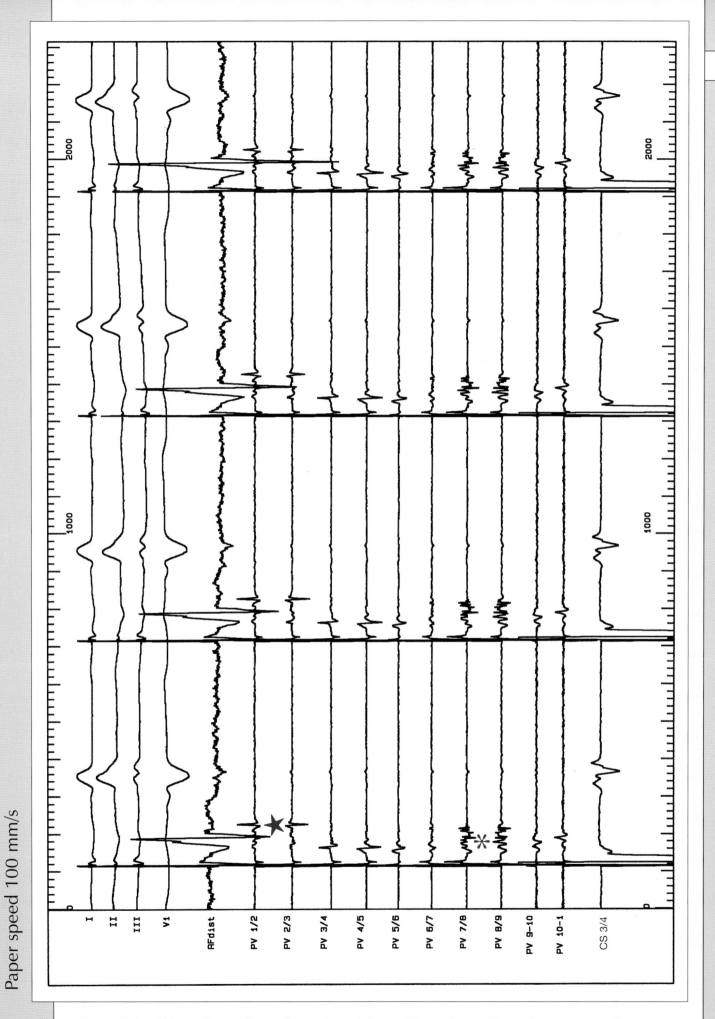

CASE 27 PART 5

- This tracing is recorded during ablation in the same vein.

  What has happened?

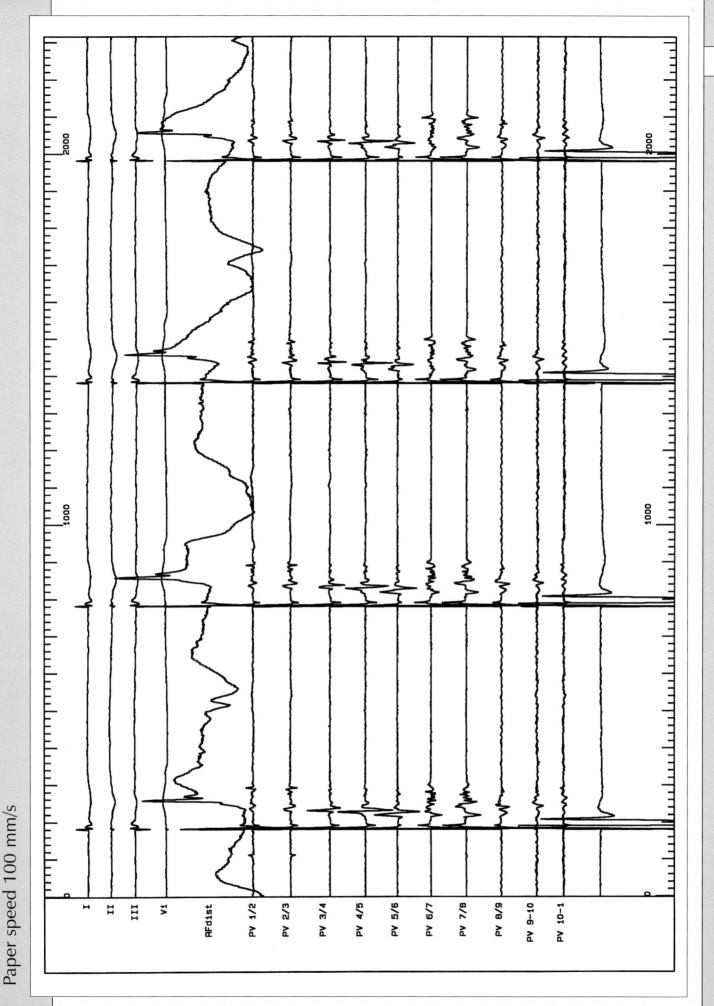

Paper speed 100 mm/s

CASE 27 PART 6

- During ablation, particularly at the posterior part of the LSPV, it is common to observe a complete AV block, most likely a vagally mediated response. Conduction quickly recovers upon cessation of energy delivery.

Paper speed 100 mm/s

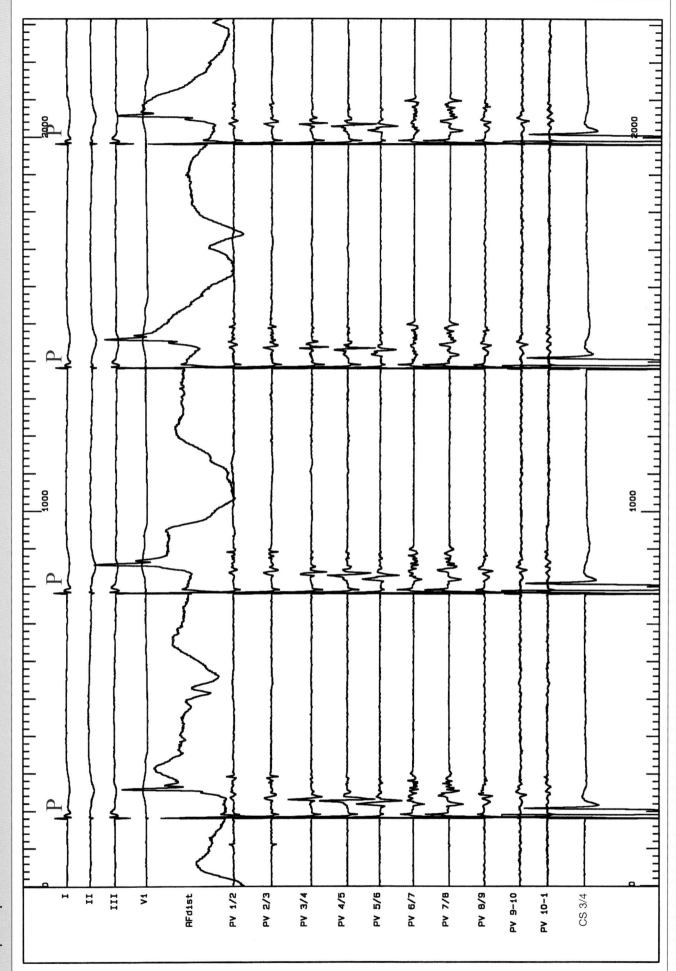

CASE 27 PART 7

- This tracing demonstrates the rapid conduction recovery upon cessation of energy delivery.

  The arrow indicates the point at which RF is stopped.

Paper speed 100 mm/s

I

II

III

V1

RFdist

PV 1/2

PV 2/3

PV 3/4

PV 4/5

PV 5/6

PV 6/7

PV 7/8

PV 8/9

PV 9-10

PV 10-1

CS 3/4

2000

1000

2000

1000

CASE 28 PART 1

- Immediately following disconnection of the left-sided PVs, a LASSO catheter was placed in the RSPV during CS pacing.

  What is your interpretation of the potentials marked by the arrows?

Paper speed 100 mm/s

221

2000

1000

2000

1000

I
II
III
V1

PV 1/2
PV 2/3
PV 3/4
PV 4/5
PV 5/6
PV 6/7
PV 7/8
PV 8/9
PV 9-10
PV 10-1

CS 3/4

CASE 28 PART 2

- In this case, all of the potentials are probably PVPs (box), with the earliest breakthrough at the top and bottom of the vein. These are the most common anatomical sites of PV breakthrough.

Paper speed 100 mm/s

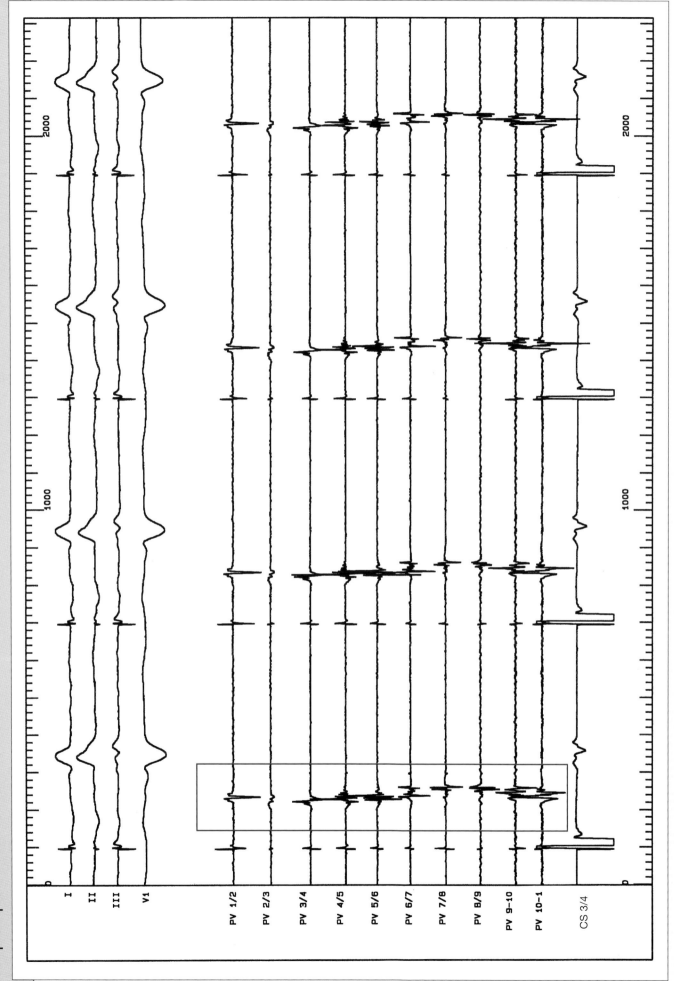

CASE 28 PART 3

- Ablation at the top of the vein (note the thermal artifact [arrows]) resulted in partial disconnection, with PVPs only remaining at the bottom.

Paper speed 100 mm/s

RF started

I

II

III

V1

RFdist

PV 1/2

PV 2/3

PV 3/4

PV 4/5

PV 5/6

PV 6/7

PV 7/8

PV 8/9

PV 9-10

PV 10-1

CS 3/4

1000

2000

1000

2000

225

- The signals of interest are late in comparison with the timing of the P wave (dotted line) in sinus rhythm, indicating either an LA origin or PVPs. They are in the posterior part of the vein, of low amplitude, and not very sharp, suggesting that they are LA far-field signals.

This can be confirmed by pacing the posterior LA near the RSPV to check whether the potentials are anticipated or delayed. If they are anticipated, they are LA far-field signals; if they are delayed, they are probably PVPs.

Paper speed 100 mm/s

Post RF

I
II
III
V1
PV 1/2
PV 2/3
PV 3/4
PV 4/5
PV 5/6
PV 6/7
PV 7/8
PV 8/9
PV 9–10
PV 10–1
CS 3/4

2000
1000

- During ablation targeting the bottom of the vein, the following were seen.

Do you think they are PVP or far-field signals?

Paper speed 100 mm/s

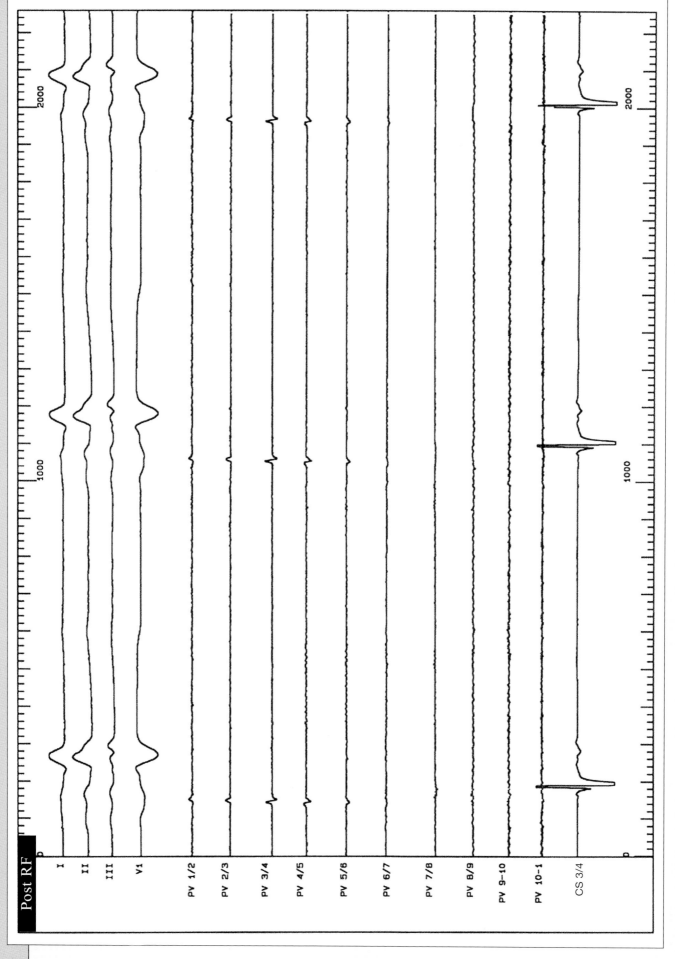

CASE 28 PART 6

- When the RSPV was disconnected, only LA far-field signals remained (A).

Paper speed 100 mm/s

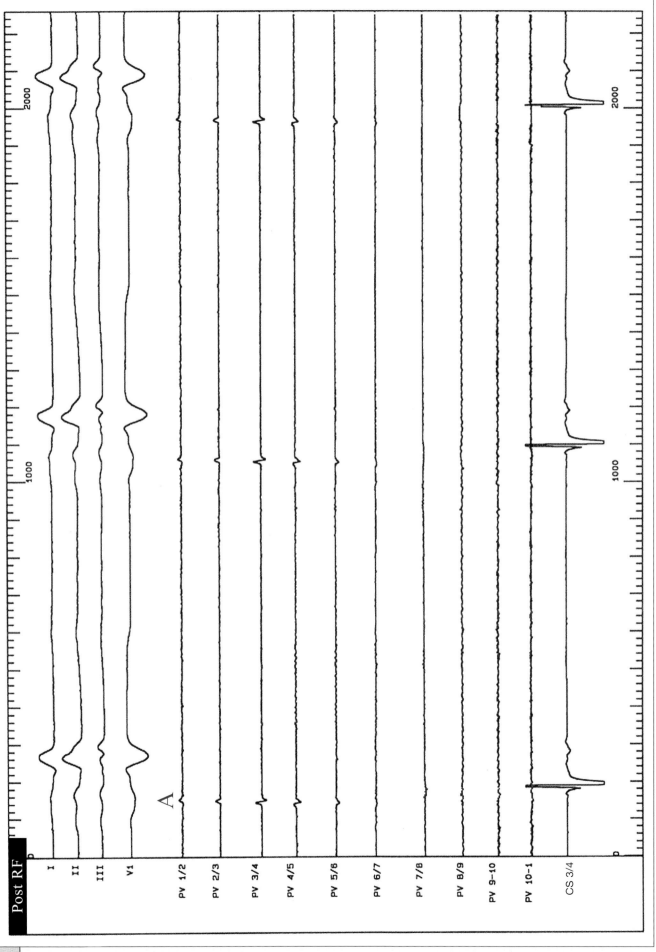

Post RF

I

II

III

V1

A

PV 1/2

PV 2/3

PV 3/4

PV 4/5

PV 5/6

PV 6/7

PV 7/8

PV 8/9

PV 9-10

PV 10-1

CS 3/4

2000

1000

2000

1000

CASE 29 PART 1

- This patient exhibited recurrence of incessant arrhythmia 24 hours after PV ablation.

  What is the probable origin of the arrhythmia?

Paper speed 25 mm/s

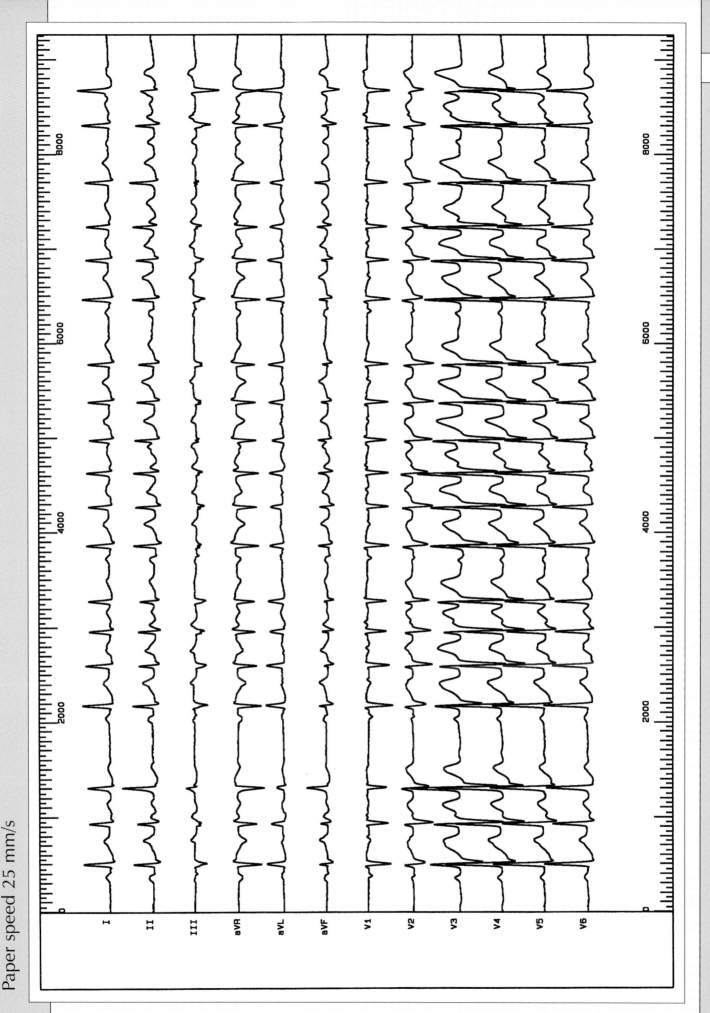

CASE 29 PART 2

- On the ECG, atrial ectopics (✳) with a positive P wave in II, III, and aVF, and aVL and I (see algorithm on page 45) suggest the diagnosis of an RSPV or right-sided LA roof origin of the arrhythmia.

Paper speed 25 mm/s

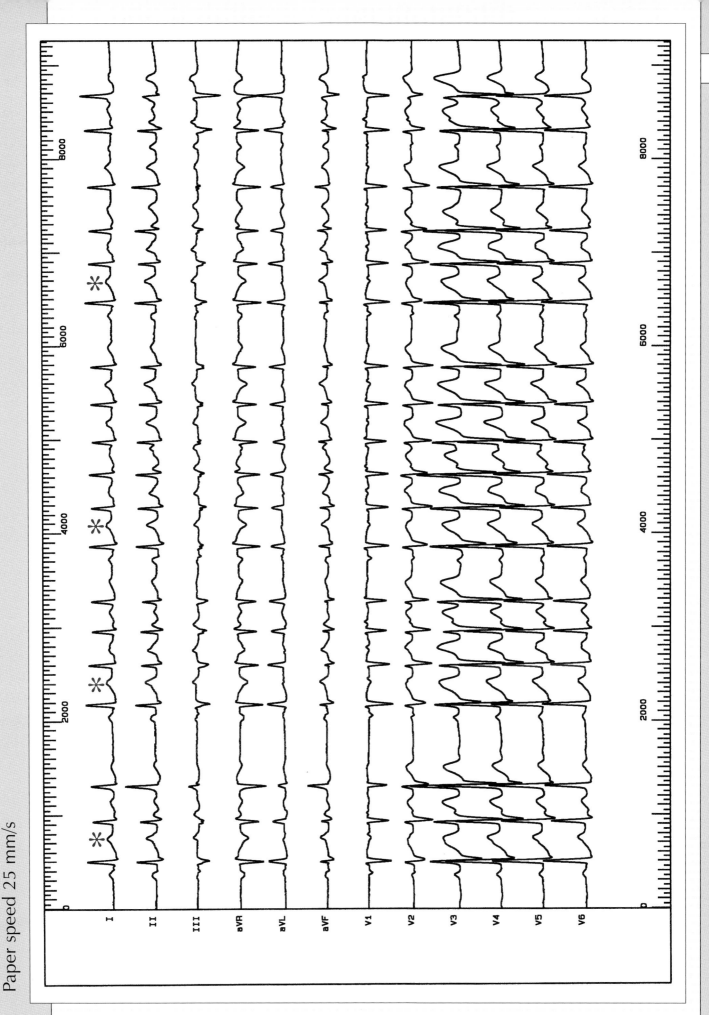

CASE 29 PART 3

- The next two tracings were recorded with the mapping catheter in different locations. In this first tracing, the mapping catheter is in the posterior LA.

Paper speed 100 mm/s

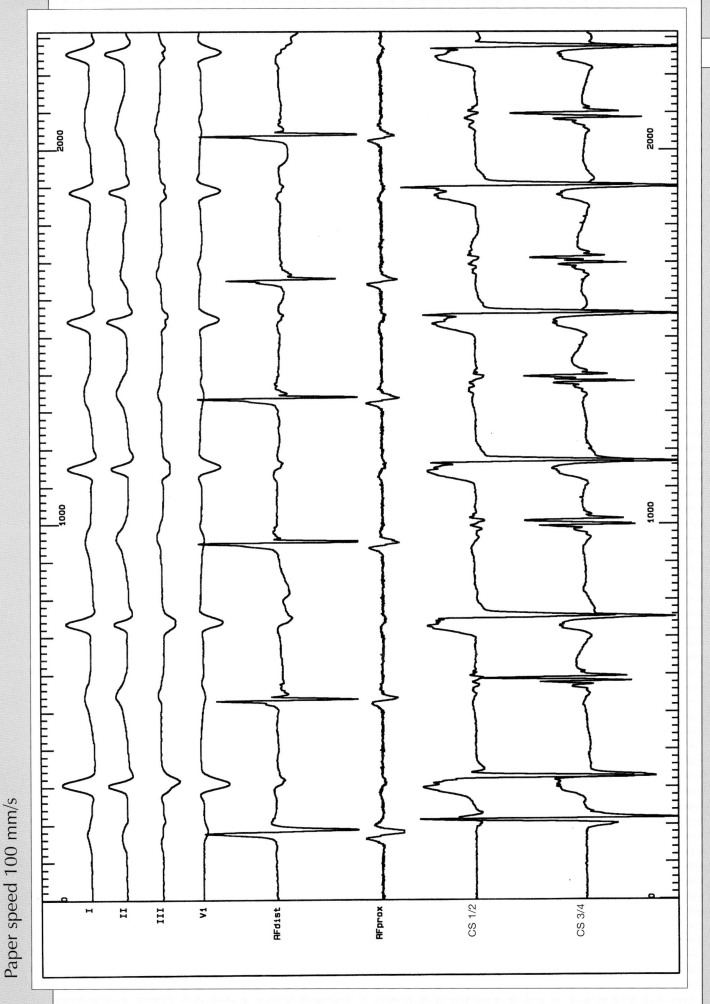

I

II

III

V1

RFdist

RFprox

CS 1/2

CS 3/4

CASE 29 PART 4

- In this second tracing, the catheter is 1 cm into the RSPV. What is the probable origin and mechanism of this arrhythmia?

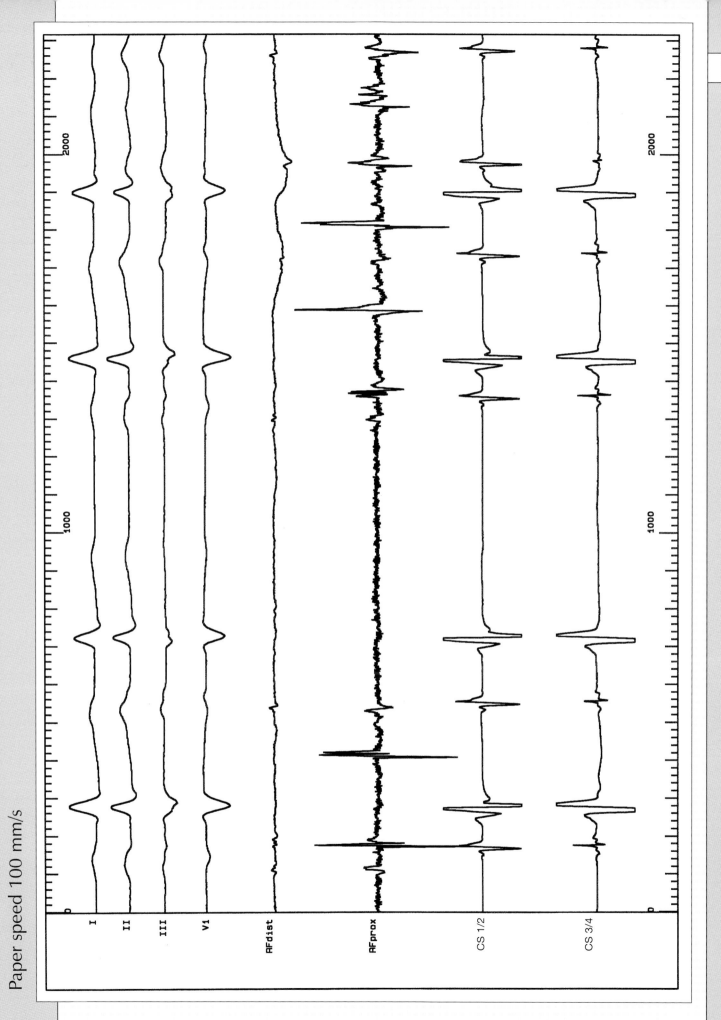

Paper speed 100 mm/s

239

CASE 29 PART 5

- Distally into the RSPV, only LA far-field signals are recorded. More proximally, at the ostium of the PV, a fragmented delayed potential (F) is recorded following atrial activation (A).

The second atrial activity recorded on this tracing corresponds to clinical ectopic beats. The origin is now visible on the map proximally. Distally, only LA far-field signals are recorded. A slight pullback of the mapping catheter more proximally will be enough to record the earliest potential and will locate the optimal ablation site (next tracing).

Paper speed 100 mm/s

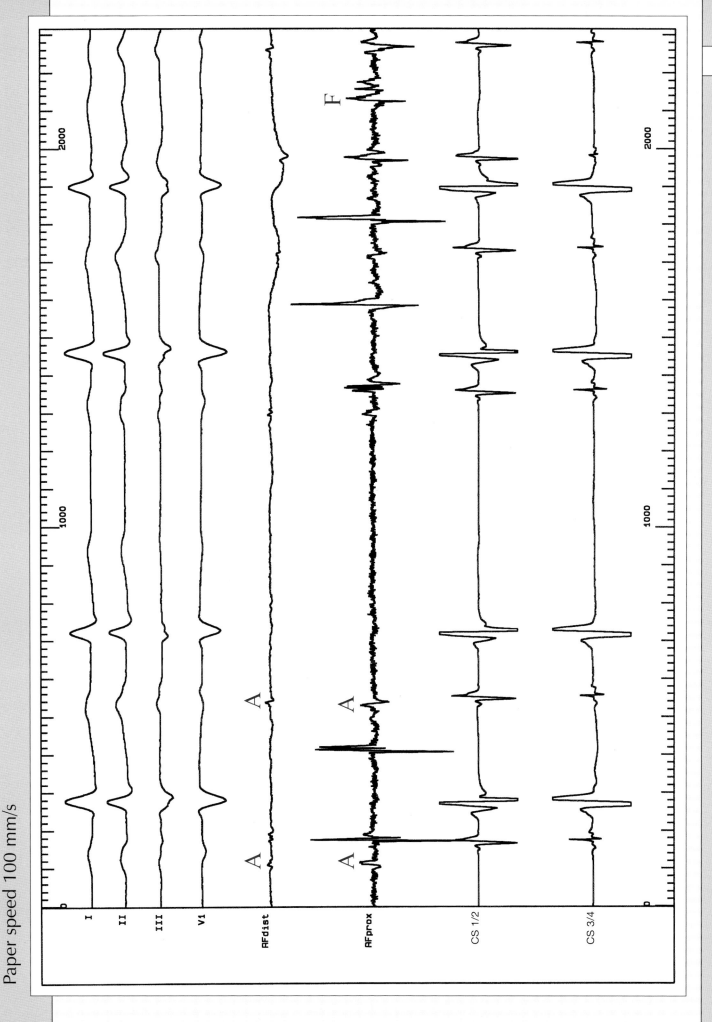

241

CASE 29 PART 6

- After pullback of the catheter towards the atrium, activation is now distal to proximal. Precocity on the P wave is maximal (dotted line). Foci in PV ostia are the most common cause of AFIB recurrence following PV disconnection.

Paper speed 100 mm/s

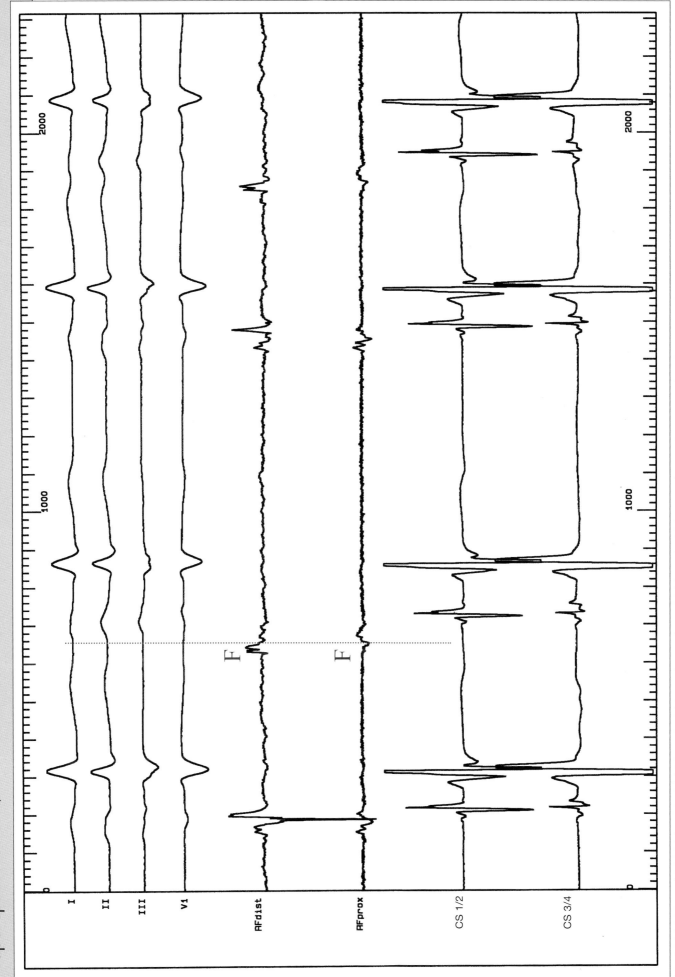

CASE 29 PART 7

- Soon after the RF ablation is started (arrow), ectopics and focal arrhythmias disappear.

Paper speed 12.5 mm/s

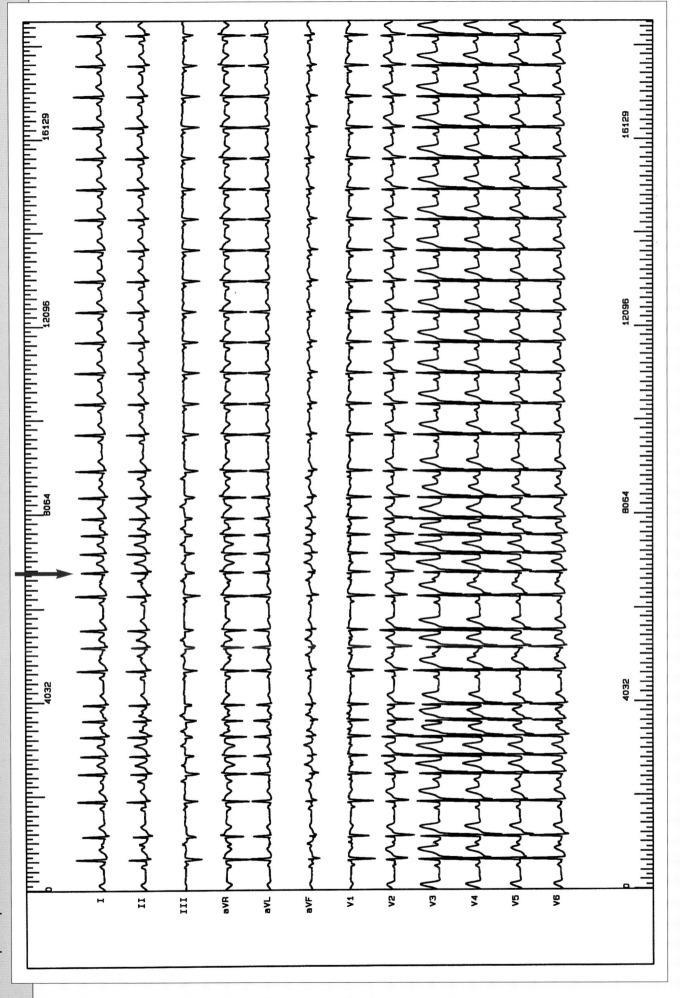

CASE 30 PART 1

- This LASSO recording is from an LSPV during AFIB (the LASSO shaft is at the top of the vein).

  Is the PV activity organized or disorganized?

Paper speed 100 mm/s

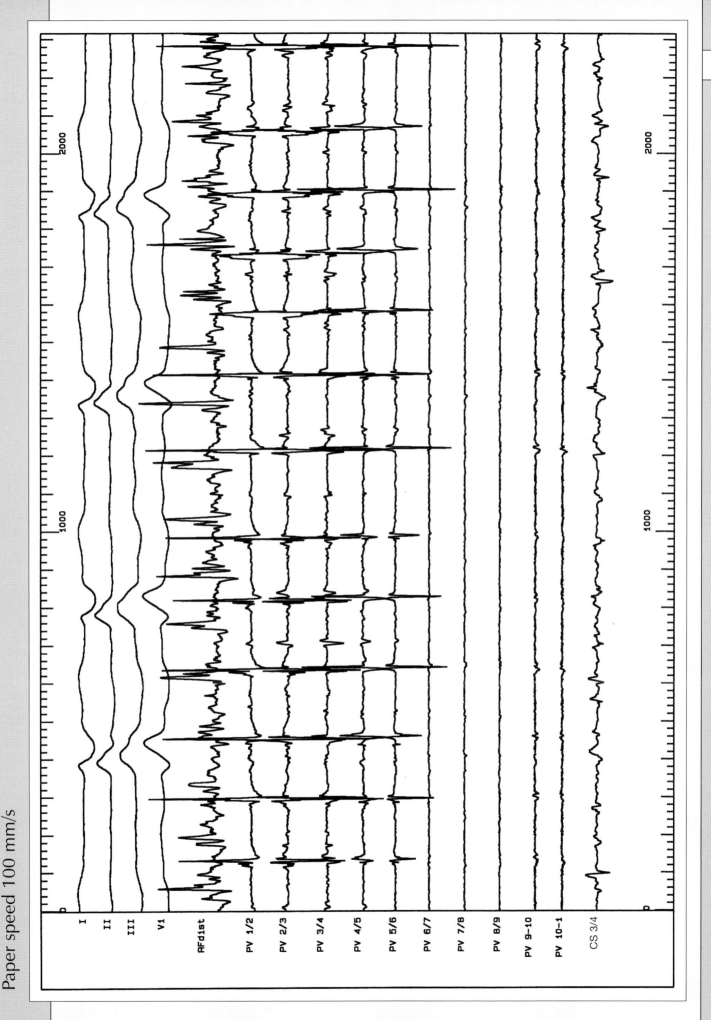

CASE 30 PART 2

- Activity within the vein is organized, with the earliest breakthrough at LASSO pole 2 (dotted line) corresponding to the top anterior part of the vein. An atrial far-field signal (A) can be seen in the anterior part of the vein.

Paper speed 100 mm/s

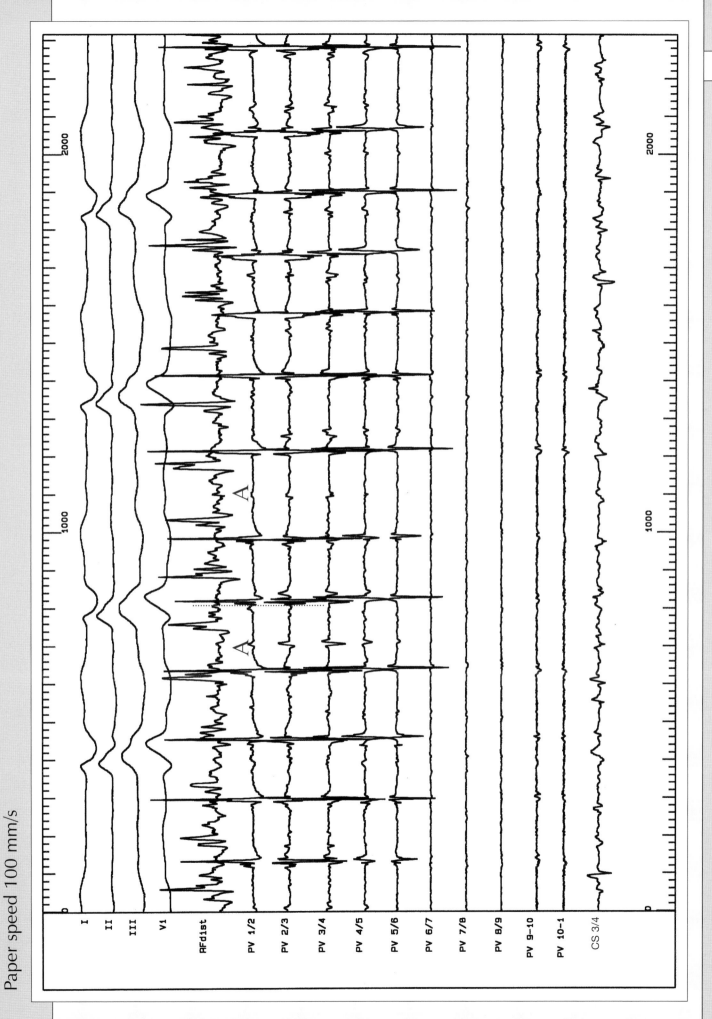

CASE 30 PART 3

- This tracing was recorded during ablation targeting LASSO pole 2.

  Would you continue ablating?

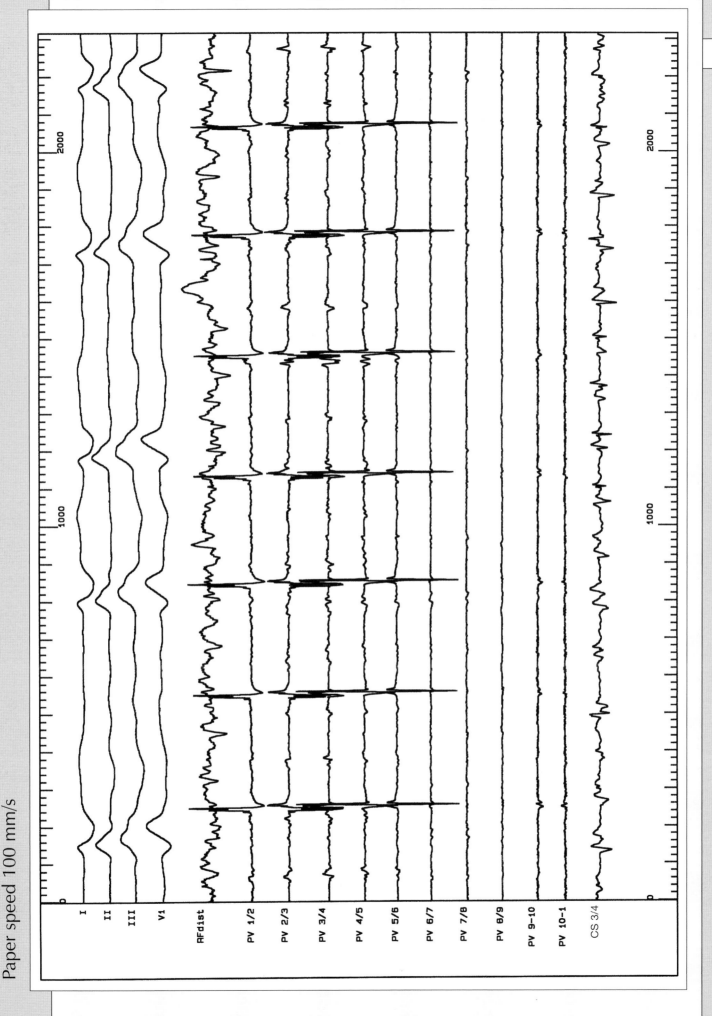

Paper speed 100 mm/s

251

CASE 30 PART 4

- This tracing shows incomplete conduction block between the LA and PV during ongoing AFIB. This phenomenon usually precedes complete disconnection, and ablation should be continued at this site.

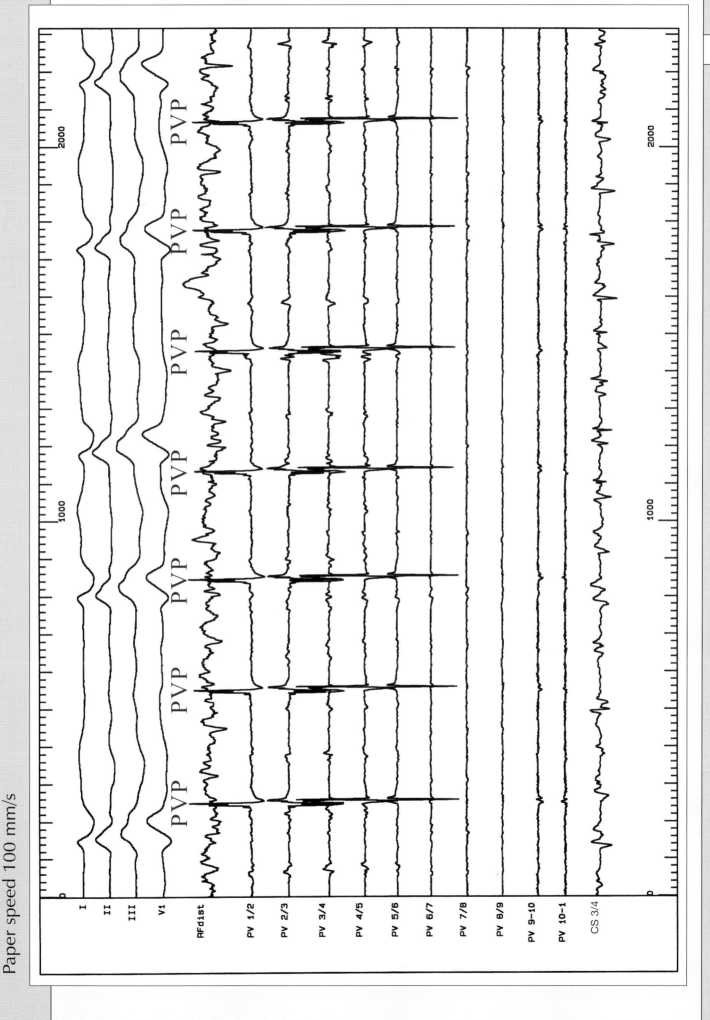

Paper speed 100 mm/s

CASE 30 PART 5

- This tracing is recorded during ongoing energy delivery.

  What has happened?

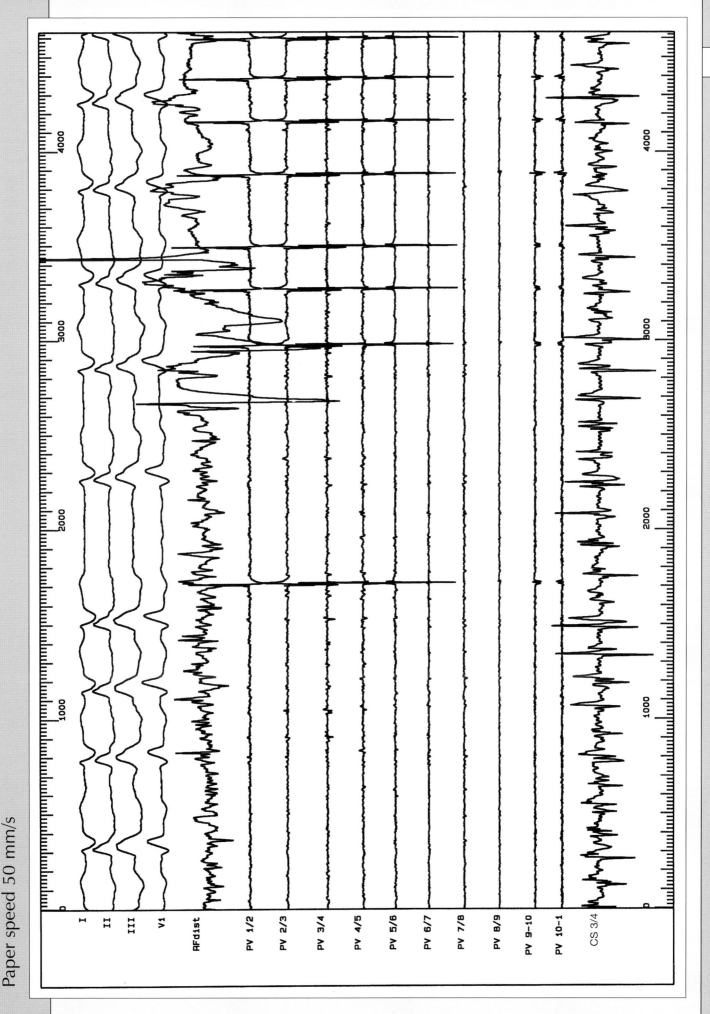

Paper speed 50 mm/s

255

CASE 30 PART 6

- The ablation catheter has moved – note the signal change (arrow) – and there is abrupt recovery of PV conduction (★). The vein was not completely disconnected prior to catheter displacement (✳). When ablating ostially, it is not uncommon for the catheter to "fall off" the ostium. This should be identified early fluoroscopically and from the local electrograms.

  This tracing also demonstrates the importance of delivering adequate energy at sites where conduction changes.

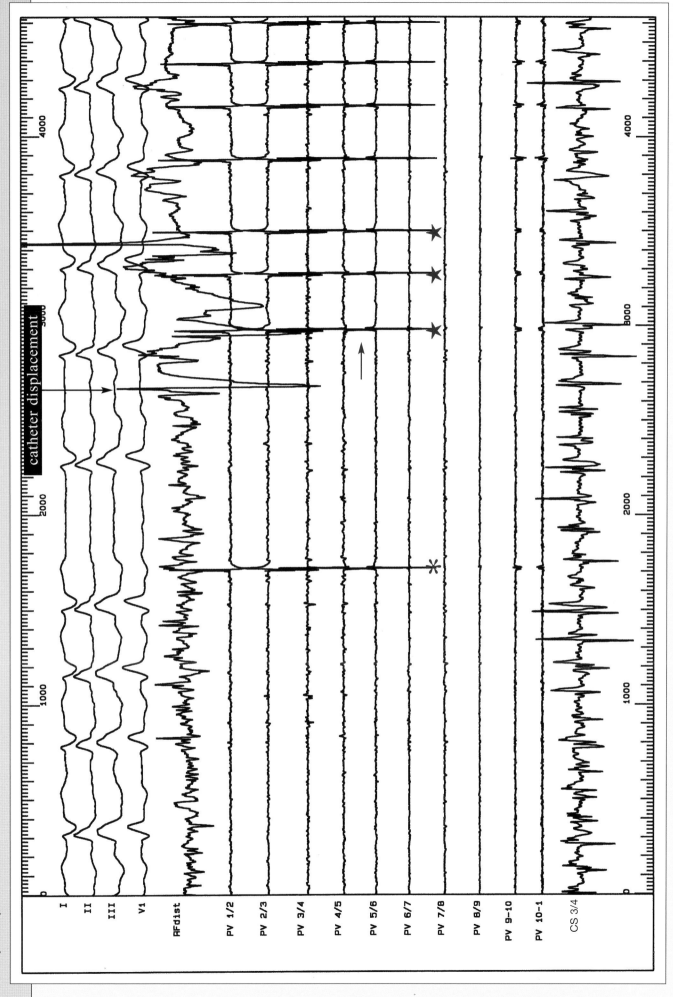

Paper speed 50 mm/s

257

CASE 31 PART 1

- This recording is from the LSPV during CS pacing after 4-PV isolation and left isthmus ablation to check that the vein is still disconnected (the LASSO shaft is at the top of the vein).

  What is your interpretation of the potentials indicated by the arrow?

Paper speed 50 mm/s

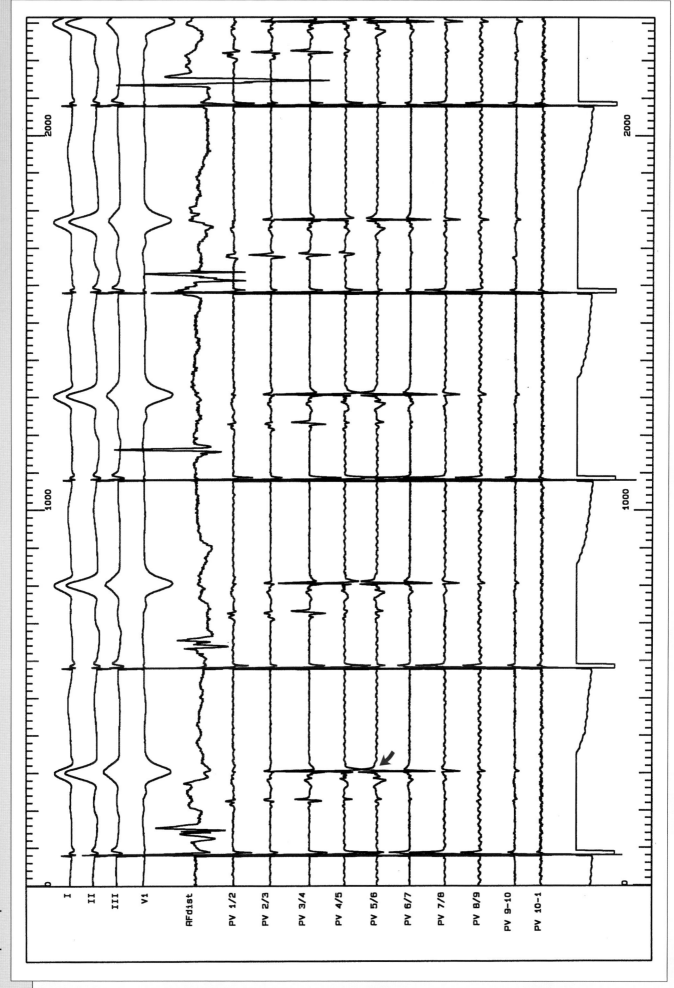

259

CASE 31 PART 2

- The potentials represent ventricular far-field signals (V) recorded from the bottom of the LIPV. There is a delay between the pacing artifact and LAA far-field signals (A) because of previous LA isthmus ablation (arrow). There is no need for further ablation within this vein.

Paper speed 50 mm/s

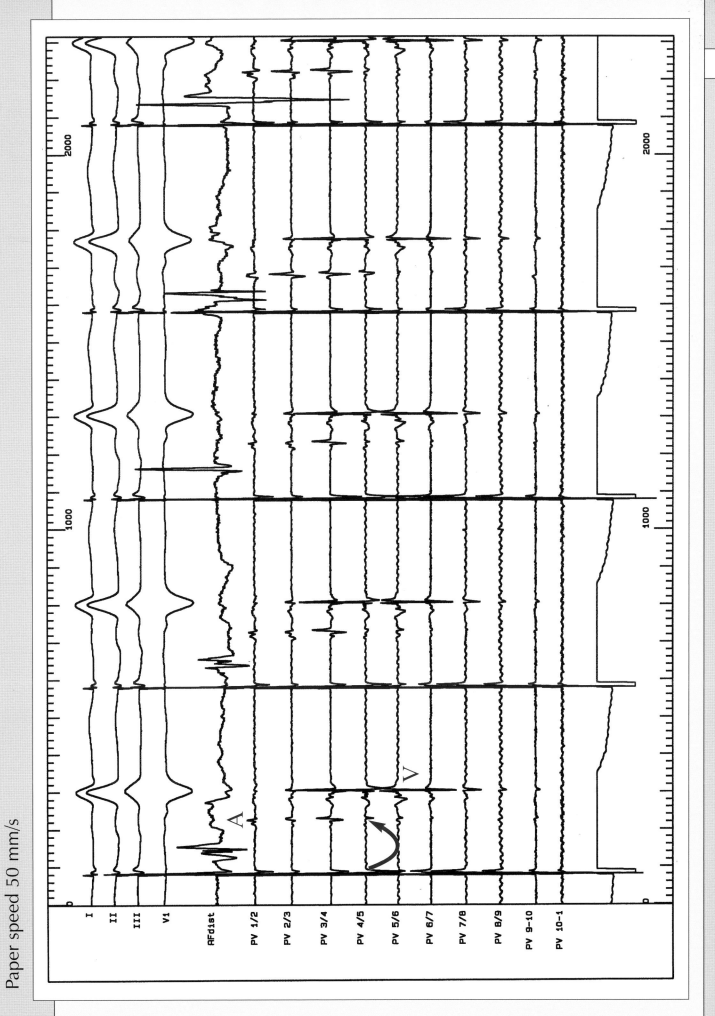

CASE 31 PART 3

- During sinus rhythm in the same patient, LAA (A) and ventricular far-field signals (V) can be appreciated.

Paper speed 100 mm/s

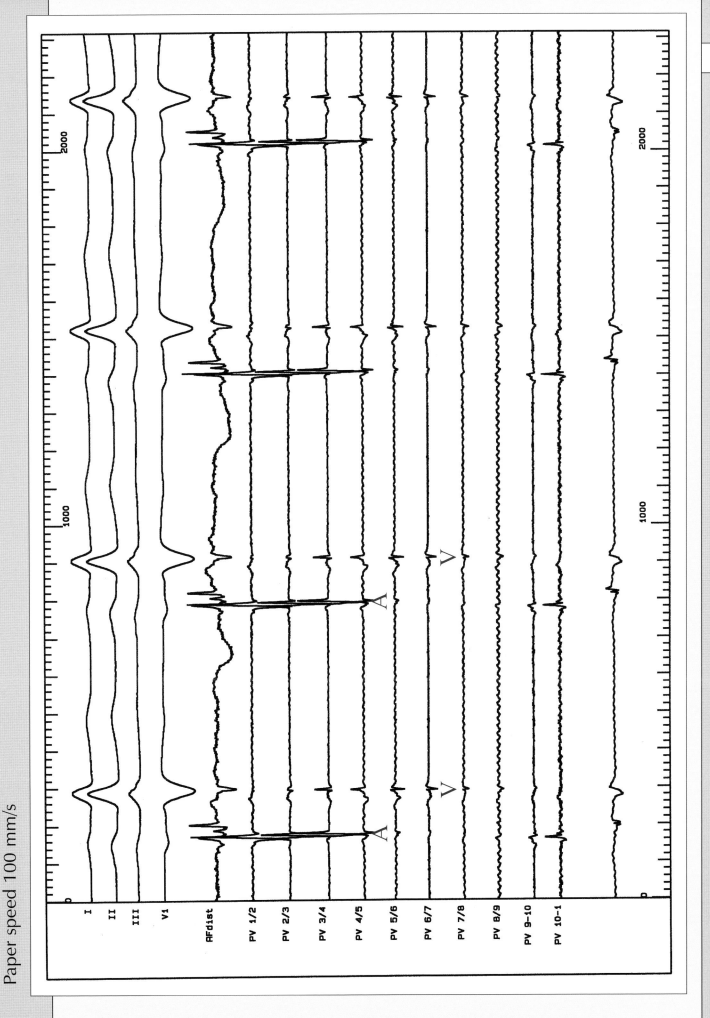

CASE 32 PART 1

- This recording is from an LSPV (the LASSO shaft is at the top of the vein) during ablation at LASSO pole 8.

  What is your interpretation?

Paper speed 100 mm/s

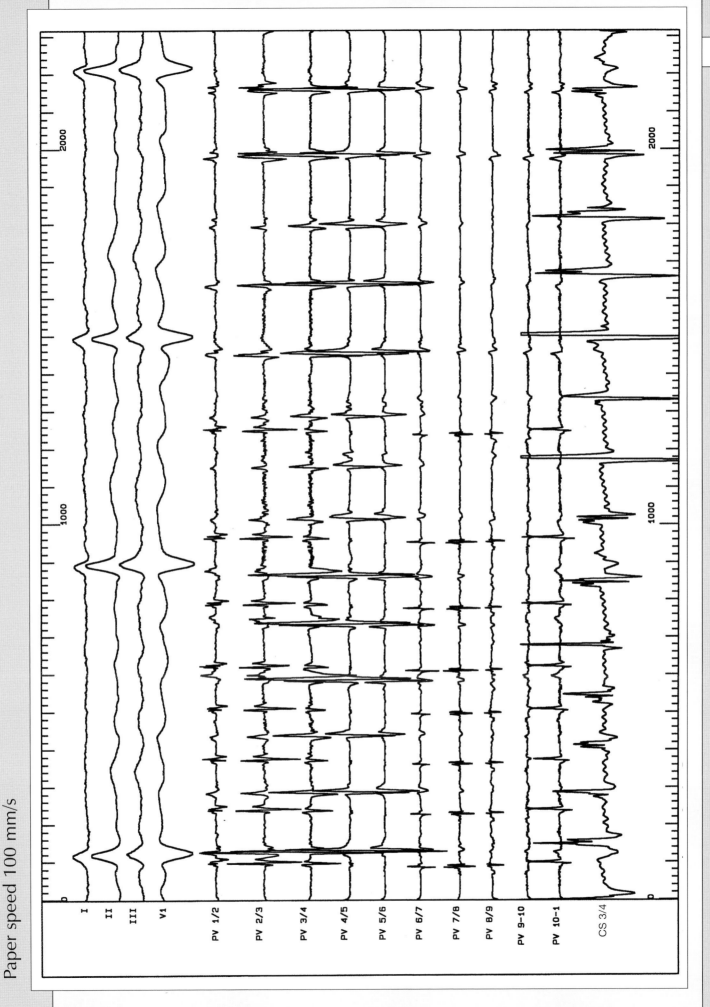

I

II

III

V1

PV 1/2

PV 2/3

PV 3/4

PV 4/5

PV 5/6

PV 6/7

PV 7/8

PV 8/9

PV 9-10

PV 10-1

CS 3/4

2000

1000

2000

1000

CASE 32 PART 2

- The tracing shows disconnection of the LSPV during ongoing AFIB. PVP (P) can be seen slowing then disappearing and all that remains are LA far-field signals (A), which are most obvious at the anterior part of the vein.

Paper speed 100 mm/s

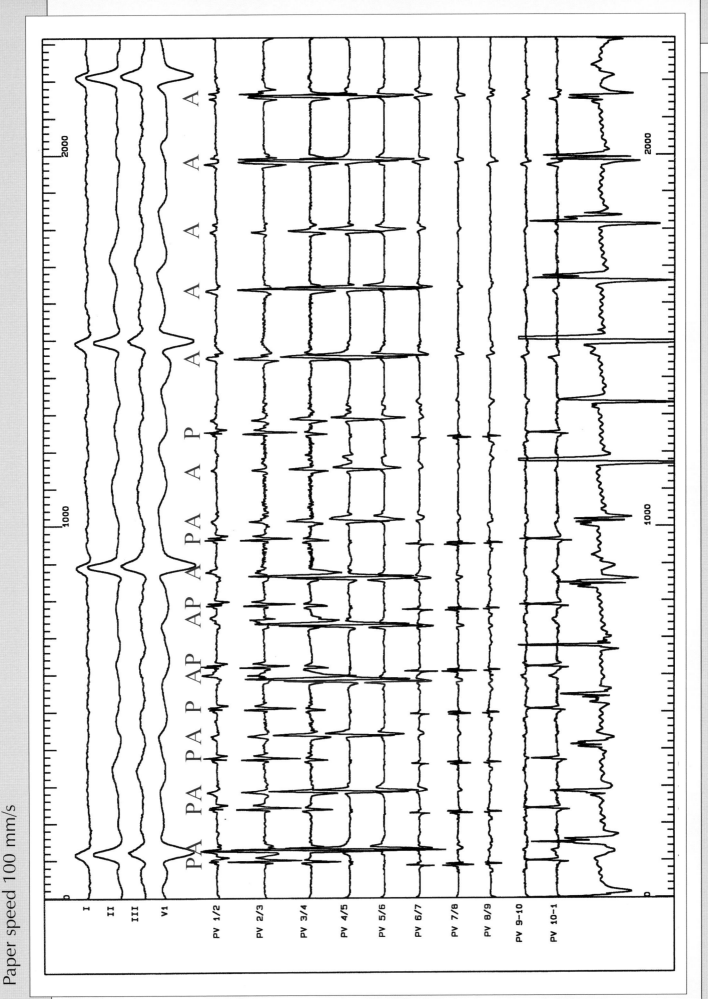

Appendices

APPENDIX 1

Navigation of the ablation catheter within the right-sided veins

- The LASSO™ shaft usually lies at the top of the vein. After entering the vein, the ablation catheter is fully curved and withdrawn to the ostium. The top of the vein is reached by de-curving the catheter. Clockwise rotation directs the catheter to the anterior wall, and counterclockwise rotation is used to reach the posterior wall.

  Ostial catheter stability can be achieved around the entire circumference of most right-sided veins, obviating the need to ablate within these veins. In contrast, in the left-sided veins, the catheter is not stable outside the vein in the anterior wall due to the presence of the left atrial appendage; therefore, ablation is performed slightly inside the vein at this site.

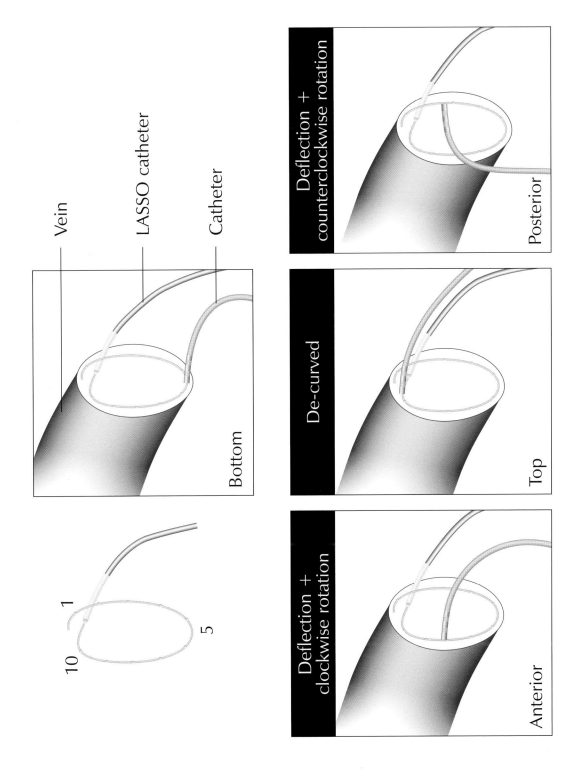

APPENDIX 2

Navigation of the mapping catheter within the left-sided veins

- The LASSO™ shaft usually lies at the top of the vein. After entering the vein, the ablation catheter is fully curved and withdrawn to the ostium. The top of the vein is reached by de-curving the catheter. Counterclockwise rotation directs the catheter to the anterior wall, and clockwise rotation is used to reach the posterior wall. When ablating the bottom and anterior wall of the left-sided veins, it is necessary to enter the vein (by a few millimeters only) to achieve catheter stability.

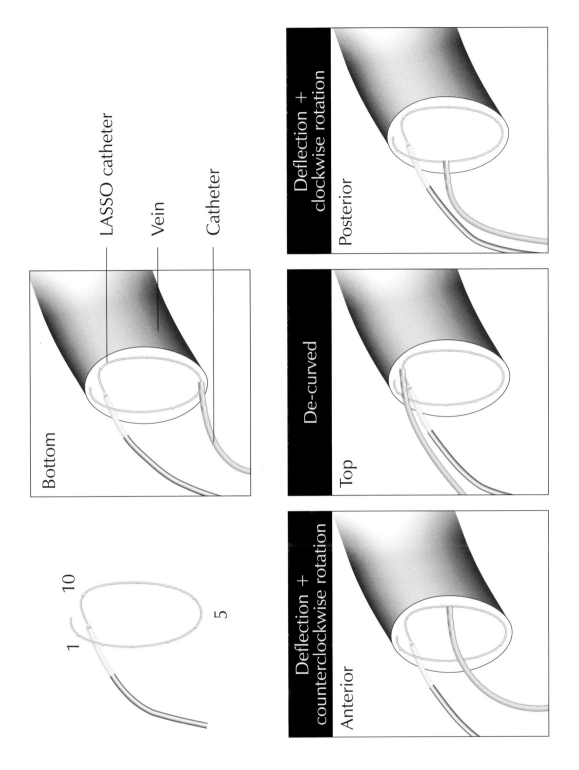

LASSO catheter

Vein

Catheter

Bottom

Deflection + clockwise rotation

Posterior

De-curved

Top

Deflection + counterclockwise rotation

Anterior

1   10

5

APPENDIX 3

Use of distal coronary sinus pacing to separate LAA and PVP in the left-sided veins

- (Top panel) During sinus rhythm, activation of the LAA and PV is almost simultaneous, resulting in fusion of LAA and PV signals on the LASSO™ recording.

- (Bottom panel) Pacing the CS changes the activation sequence so that the LAA is activated first (light red signals) and the PV second (dark red signals). This results in clear separation of the signals on the LASSO recording.

Further reading

Shah D, Haissaguerre M, Jais P, Hocini M, Yamane T, Macle L, Choi KJ, Clementy J. Left atrial appendage activity masquerading as pulmonary vein potentials. *Circulation* 2002;105:2821–5.

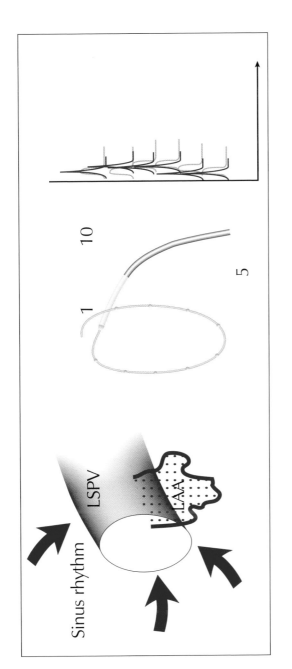

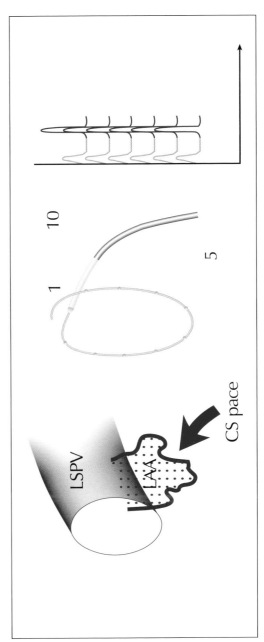

APPENDIX 4

Polarity reversal

- (Top panel) Polarity reversal refers to the PVP pattern depicted in black. One PV spike is predominantly positive, while the contiguous PV spike is predominantly negative.

- (Bottom panel) The mechanism of polarity reversal. At points of LA to PV breakthrough, polarity reversal of the PV signal is recorded by the LASSO™ catheter as the wavefront disperses in two opposing directions. Therefore, polarity reversal can be used to determine breakthrough in cases where there is doubt or if there is no clear PVP cascade.

Further reading

Yamane T, Shah DC, Jais P, Hocini M M, Deisenhofer I, Choi KJ, Macle L, Clementy J, Haissaguerre M. Electrogram polarity reversal as an additional indicator of breakthroughs from the left atrium to the pulmonary veins. *J Am Coll Cardiol* 2002;39:1337–44.

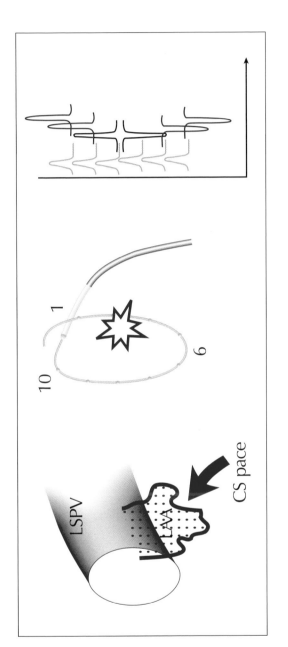

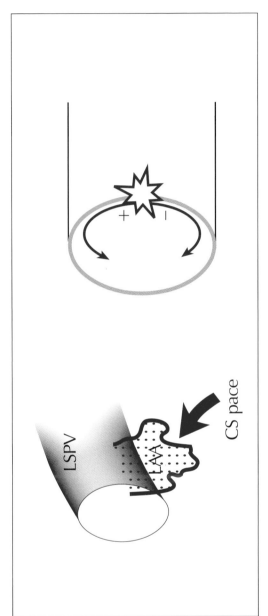

APPENDIX 5

Explanation of PVP patterns during atrial fibrillation

- (Top panel) When there are multiple LA to PV connections the pattern is disorganized, because different parts of the PV circumference are activated in a random manner.

- (Bottom panel) The pattern is organized if there are limited PV breakthroughs, because electrical activity in the atrium must be filtered through the remaining fascicles to enter the PV.

Further reading

Macle L, Jais P, Scavee C, Weerasooriya R, Shah DC, Hocini M, Choi KJ, Raybaud F, Clementy J, Haissaguerre M. Electrophysiologically guided pulmonary vein isolation during sustained atrial fibrillation. *J Cardiovasc Electrophysiol* 2003;14:255–60.

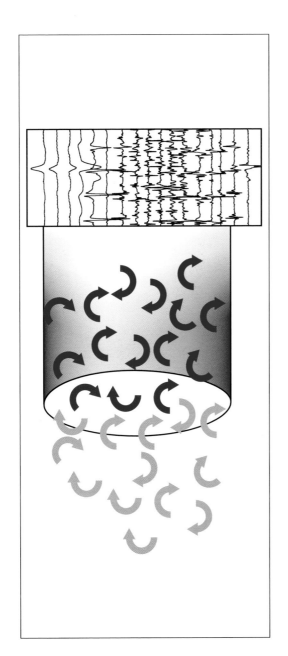
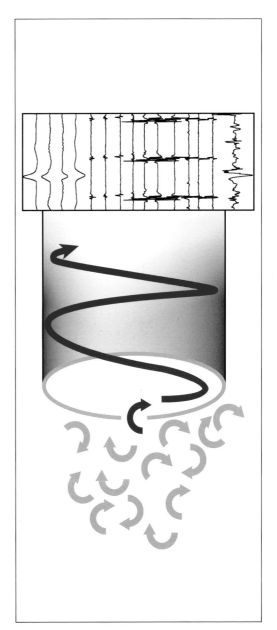